Hormone Replacement T~~~

Hormone Replacement Therapy

Making Your Own Decision

PATSY WESTCOTT

Thorsons
An Imprint of HarperCollins*Publishers*

Thorsons
An Imprint of HarperCollins*Publishers*
77–85 Fulham Palace Road,
Hammersmith, London W6 8JB

Published by Thorsons 1993
10 9 8 7 6 5 4 3 2 1

A catalogue record for this book
is available from the British Library

ISBN 0 7225 2782 9

Typeset by Harper Phototypesetters Limited,
Northampton, England
Printed in Great Britain by
The Guernsey Press Co. Ltd, Guernsey, Channel Islands

Contents

Acknowledgements

The author would like to thank the women whose experiences make up the case histories described in this book. The words are their own, but their names have been changed to protect their privacy.

Preface

The Times They Are A-Changin'

Just over a hundred years ago, our great-grandmothers couldn't expect to live much beyond the age of 40; by the beginning of this century, life expectancy had gone up to 55 years. Today we can expect to go on to the ripe old age of 80. In 1992 there are almost 10 million women over the age of 50 in the UK. By the year 2029 there will be 12.5 million – more than a fifth of the total population. Never before have there been so many post-menopausal women, and never before have so many opportunities been open to them.

In our great-grandmothers' time women who were lucky enough to survive the ordeal of childbirth had no choice but to accept the slowing down and ill-health that were regarded as inevitable in 'old age'. By contrast, women approaching the menopause today can look forward to three decades or more of healthy, active life untroubled by the discomforts of periods, pre-menstrual tension, and pregnancy.

That's the good news. The bad is that the menopause can create a range of health problems which if not tackled may result in a poorer quality of life.

The profile of the menopausal woman is changing, too. The housewife whose children were moving away from home, leaving her with an 'empty nest', is giving way to the busy, working mother, struggling to juggle the demands of home and work. With the increasing tendency for women to delay having children until their 30s and even 40s, in favour of developing their careers, a whole generation of women are about to hit the menopause who are very different from previous generations.

I am a member of this 'new' generation. Many of us still have young children to care for and jobs to hold down. Many others are divorced or separated, or are single parents with all these responsibilities; some are embarking on new relationships and careers. We expect and feel we deserve to be in tip-top health.

But as we approach the menopause, many of us do so with a sense of apprehension. What can we expect? Will the menopause transform us, as some accounts seem to threaten, from vital, energetic individuals into lack-lustre old crones? Or will it be, as others promise, a time of liberation when we can at last grow and develop in ways that are not dictated by other people? And what about Hormone Replacement Therapy (HRT)? Can it fend off the misery of hot sweats, save our sex lives, and protect us against the menopausal depression? Even more intriguing, will it stave off ageing and keep us looking young and beautiful? Or will we all die of breast cancer before we reach our sixtieth birthday?

We are the Pill pioneers. The contraceptive Pill gave us choice, freedom from the necessity of childbearing, control over our biological destiny. But in the light of some of the question marks being raised, many of us are wondering whether we will have to pay too high a price for our freedom. Many of us are wary of chemical solutions, and have become interested in exploring alternative therapies to help ourselves live healthy lives. Yet we wonder, will our bodies let us down?

HRT holds out the promise of freeing us from the miseries many of us dread, yet at the same time we are afraid. Will this too turn out to be a bitter Pill? We try to get information, only to be faced with confusion and contradiction. We are not helped by the fact that all too many of those we turn to for advice have vested interests of one sort or another.

In this book I attempt to look honestly at these questions, to examine the pros and cons of HRT, and to put some of the issues into perspective. What I discovered was that, despite the reams written about the subject, it is *still* difficult to get the facts about HRT. As a specialist health writer and journalist who has often written about childbirth, I found myself facing a familiar scenario. The menopause, like pregnancy and childbirth, has been turned into an illness.

Yet at the same time there is a serious lack of real choice and facilities for menopausal women. Those who consult their doctors for help and reassurance are often met with ignorance, lack of interest or a confusion that mirrors their own. On the other hand, those who do opt for medical help sometimes feel they have simply been put on an HRT production line. Others go on the therapy but somehow feel they have failed, that if they had possessed enough moral fibre they would have struggled stoically on. The fact is there still aren't enough menopause clinics, and those that do exist don't always offer any real choice. We need more well-woman clinics. But we also need to take responsibility for ourselves so that we can make sure that these clinics offer us a truly holistic health service that takes into account our individual needs.

I hope I have given a balanced view of both the risks and benefits of HRT based on what is known at the moment. I have also included hints on self-help and alternative therapies that you may want to explore to help make sure you are fit for the menopause.

Let's make sure that the times are changing for the better.

PATSY WESTCOTT, 1993

Introduction

HRT ~ Curse or Cure?

'I was dizzy, my memory went to pot, my skin dried up and my hair started coming out. I thought I was going senile. It came as a complete shock to me because I'd never had any women's problems. I'd always kept fit and eaten a good diet; I didn't expect to be so thrown by the menopause. My sex life was affected too. I got so dry I didn't want to know, and I kept getting cystitis.

   'Fortunately my doctor was sympathetic and referred me to a menopause clinic where I was prescribed HRT. When I first went on it I got painful calves and tender breasts, but gradually these settled down and now I feel wonderful. My feeling of well-being came back within a month. My memory is as good as it was and I can enjoy life again. And a lot of people remark I look younger.'

JUDITH, 45

'My periods began to be irregular from when I was 38. Then when I was 42 I remember feeling dizzy and having a funny turn at work. After that the flushes and sweats started and I became ratty. The doctor put me on HRT for three months, but when I went back I saw a woman doctor who thought it was too soon for the menopause, so she took me off. All the symptoms returned. It ruined one holiday in Tenerife. I was sweating all the time. At the end of that time my doctor decided it *was* the menopause, and she put me on HRT again for 12 months. At first it was OK, but then I began to get terrible trouble with my legs and feet. I also developed bad headaches. I felt like a zombie. I would open my mouth to speak and a load of gibberish would come out. In the end I decided to try homoeopathy.

'The sweats gradually stopped and I got my brain back. I was able to make decisions. One of the first was to give up my job. Now I am enjoying life again, spending time with my family, which I didn't have time to do before, and enjoying my grandson. I tried HRT once more, because I have a history of osteoporosis [brittle bone disease] in my family. But the minute I went back on it all the old problems recurred. I didn't want to bother with people and I became tearful. I'm now going for a bone scan: if it shows I am at risk of osteoporosis, I will have to think about what I want to do, but I definitely won't be going back on HRT – it didn't suit me.'

RUTH, 45

Two women, two experiences of HRT, but as these two accounts show the therapy arouses strong opinions and emotions. These range from the evangelical zeal of devotees such as MP Teresa Gorman – whose crusade to put HRT on the agenda has done much to foster current interest in the treatment – to the rage and condemnation of the therapy and the way it is marketed, expressed in Germaine Greer's book *The Change*.

Both women in their separate ways have raised the profile of HRT and created recognition of the special needs of menopausal women. For many women going through or approaching the change of life, however, there is still confusion. The extreme views of the zealots on both sides have raised more questions than answers. Is HRT 'the most important advance in preventive medicine in the Western world,' as claimed by gynaecologist John Studd, one of the pioneers of HRT? Or is it part and parcel of a campaign designed by drug companies, aided and abetted by doctors, to persuade us to take their products?

Doctors share in the confusion. Ruth's story is typical: different doctors had different views, and despite the fact that she was experiencing menopausal symptoms, one of her doctors took her off the therapy, with the result that she suffered a rebound which ruined her holiday. Survey after survey confirms that many doctors are ill-informed and unsure when it comes to prescribing HRT. One such survey, carried out in the spring of 1992 by National Opinion Polls for the drug company Ciba-Geigy, showed that only two thirds of respondents considered their doctors a useful source of information about the menopause and HRT. Another survey, for the magazine *Woman's Realm*, carried out in conjunction with HRT manufacturer Schering, reported that doctors didn't know enough about the different varieties of HRT on offer. A third independent survey, performed by nurse Joyce Masling and reported in *Nursing Times* (September 1988), found that one third of women were dissatisfied with their doctors, whom they found unsympathetic.

Behind the inconsistent prescribing patterns, lack of information and confusion there lie some real concerns. Above all there is fear: that by taking HRT we are somehow tampering with Nature, and that in so doing we are storing up trouble for ourselves in the future. These fears were summed up by the woman who confided, 'I can't quite put my finger on it, I just feel instinctively that it's not a good thing to be stuffing yourself with hormones.' The experts argue that such worries are irrational, a result of ignorance and lack of knowledge about the true facts. None the less, they deserve to be taken seriously.

The problem is that all the pronouncements, news stories, scares and counterscares make it extremely hard for anyone –

medically trained or otherwise – to evaluate HRT and decide whether it makes sense. Judging by regular reports in the papers about the risks of HRT, you might be forgiven for wondering why any woman should choose to take it. *Yet few therapies have the potential to do so much good – prevention of heart disease and osteoporosis – or so much harm – boosting the risk of breast cancer – as HRT.*

In this book I attempt to cut through the hype of both the proponents and opponents and bring you the facts so you can make up your own mind whether HRT is right for you. But first let's trace the story of HRT, through the pages of the press.

The Irresistible Rise (and Fall and Rise) of HRT

HRT, like its sister drug the contraceptive Pill, has attracted controversy ever since it first hit the headlines back in the 1960s. The sixties were the decade when faith in technology and the power of the 'magic bullet' was at its strongest.

The story of HRT is a fascinating one because it mirrors the rise and fall of our belief in modern medicine. The recent resurgence in popularity of HRT, together with a more questioning approach to the treatment and its side-effects, marks a more realistic awareness that every treatment has costs as well as benefits. It is also a story that highlights the powerful yet double-edged role the press plays in informing us about new advances in medicine. Today we are perhaps more sceptical of the reports we read in the papers, realizing that at best they offer only a partial account of medical developments.

Back in 1966, however, when Brooklyn doctor Robert Wilson's book *Forever Feminine* was published, HRT was greeted effusively. Wilson listed no less than 26 different symptoms that could be attributed to the menopause. 'No woman can be sure of escaping the horror of this living decay,' he warned emotively.

'Menopause is one of nature's mistakes,' declared Dr Joseph W. Goldzieher in a 1967 *Newsweek* article devoted to the runaway success of Wilson's book. The same article went on to explain that the menopause was a deficiency disease in much the same way as diabetes – an argument still advanced today. Wilson claimed that four out of ten women between 35 and 40 were already oestrogen-deficient, and that nine out of ten would be within four or five years of stopping menstruating. He advised all women to have a routine annual cervical smear from the age of 17, which would provide what he called a 'Femininity Index' – a somewhat loaded term used to describe the level of oestrogen in a woman's body.

Women with a drop in oestrogen levels were prescribed HRT – oestrogen pills to boost these levels and return them to 'normal'. These pills were taken for three weeks a month, then discontinued to produce a period during the fourth week. Interestingly enough, Wilson also prescribed an early form of HRT as we know it today – oestrogen with progestogen (the synthetic form of the naturally-occurring hormone progesterone) to be taken during the last ten days of the 21-day pill-taking period – in order to avoid the build-up of the lining of the uterus that is now known to cause cancer. However, many doctors prescribed just oestrogen alone.

The claims being made for HRT then are familiar to anyone who has followed recent news stories. The *Newsweek* article continued, 'Advocates of [HRT] believe that the treatment stops the development of osteoporosis . . . And they are convinced that the treatment . . . *makes a woman feel younger*, eliminating hot [flushes] and depression.' [My italics.]

Even in those halcyon days, some medics sounded a note of caution. Dr Edmund R. Novak of Johns Hopkins, also quoted in the *Newsweek* article, was more moderate in his approach, believing that only 5 to 10 per cent of women needed to be prescribed the treatment on a temporary basis for the relief of symptoms such as hot flushes. However, Novak's dismissal of the problems of menopausal women as 'psychological – a concern, for example, about the superficialities of looks – rather than physical' did nothing to address the very real concerns of women going through the physical and emotional

17

upheavals of the change of life.

With characteristic caution women in the UK never jumped on the HRT bandwagon with quite the same unabashed enthusiasm as their sisters across the Atlantic – by 1968 only a quarter of a million British women were taking the drug, compared with 10 million in America. But HRT continued quietly to gain in popularity. In 1972 the charity Women's Health Care (now Women's Health Concern) was set up, with backing from the drug company Ayrst, to promote the benefits of HRT. In 1975 Wendy Cooper published the first edition of her book *No Change: A Biological Revolution for Women*. The high-spot came in 1975 when the German drug company Schering launched the product *Progynova* to ecstatic press coverage: the *Daily Mail* hailed it as the 'Happiness Pill'.

But as with any newspaper saga, what goes up must come down, and later the same year the first alarm bells started to ring: a disturbing number of women on oestrogen in the US were found to have developed cancer of the endometrium – the lining of the womb. In one of the studies the risk rate varied from 5.6 to 13.7 depending on the length of oestrogen use. In another the risk was 4.5 however long the therapy was used. In the same year the first report linking HRT with an increase in the risk of breast cancer also appeared. Yet another study carried out by Macclesfield doctor Dr Jean Coope showed that women on a particular type of HRT had an increased tendency to blood clotting which suggested that the drug – like the Pill – might increase the risk of diseases such as stroke and coronary heart failure. The honeymoon was over.

With ten million women in the States on oestrogen replacement therapy, the FDA (Food and Drug Administration) ordered an immediate enquiry.

Subsequent investigation revealed that many of the early studies were flawed. Firstly, they were retrospective – i.e. looking back at records. Secondly, the doses taken by the women were not spelled out, and thirdly, it wasn't clear whether the women had taken the combined form of HRT – with the addition of progestogen to produce a monthly 'period' or shedding of the lining of the womb – or continuously as oestrogen alone. An item in the *Sunday Times* (September 1978) reported that 80 per cent of the British women taking HRT were taking it in the outdated, continuous form.

Further research confirmed that unopposed oestrogen, i.e. oestrogen taken without a balancing dose of progesterone, did indeed raise the risk of endometrial cancer. Today all women on HRT who have not had a hysterectomy have to take this balancing dose of progesterone to prevent dangerous build-up of the womb lining.

In the more sober 1970s, in the light of these and other worrying reports, a more questioning approach came into play. In a letter to the medical journal the *Lancet* (April 1977), gynaecologist James Owen Drife wrote: 'Certain pharmaceutical firms have started an energetic campaign to alter our view of menopausal women. Using film shows, glossy handouts, and lavish hospitality they are trying to persuade doctors that being a woman and over 50 is a disease, susceptible to "treatment" with oestrogens.'

In the 1980s there was a resurgence of interest in HRT with the development of new, more sophisticated formulations designed to overcome the earlier problems. Glamorous American and British actresses such as Jane Fonda, Jill Gascoigne and *Dynasty*'s Kate O'Mara publicly supported it. Both Mrs Thatcher and the Queen were rumoured to be on it. A report by medical journalist Christine Doyle in the *Daily Telegraph* (January 1989) stated the view of 'one doctor who prescribes HRT to many women in the public eye,' saying he 'would be very surprised if women who were prominent in public life did not take it.'

But no sooner had HRT begun to rise in popularity than the clouds began to gather again. A worrying Swedish report in the prestigious *New England Journal of Medicine* showed that women who had been prescribed HRT for an average of six years had an increased risk of breast cancer. And the longer they took the treatment, the greater their risk. In statistical terms the risk was slight – an increase in the odds of contracting the disease from two to three per thousand – but in view of the high risk of breast cancer that exists in the West (1 in 12 women will contract it at some time), still enough to cause many women to ask, 'Is it worth it?'

This time the progestogen component of HRT also came under scrutiny, because of the possibility that it might reduce some of oestrogen's preventive effects against heart attack and stroke. Malcolm Pike, professor of preventive medicine at the University of Southern California, quoted in a feature in the *Times* (1989), summed up the problem like this: 'For each cancer you cause with HRT, you will save six deaths from hip fractures, heart disease and stroke. In absolute terms it saves lives.' Pike himself questioned whether the progestogen component was worth adding. But he added, 'It may be many years before we get the full picture. However, on the results we have now, the balance of risk is favourable towards HRT.'

The next big scare came in February 1992, when it was reported that some women using HRT implants and patches had become dependent on high doses of oestrogen, causing them to return for repeat doses at ever-more-frequent intervals. Under the headline, 'HRT Can Be as Addictive as Heroin', the *Times* quoted psychiatrists Thomas and Susan Bewley as saying, 'One has to remember that heroin, cocaine, amphetamines, bromides, barbiturates and opiates were initially regarded as safe.' Interviewed in the *Daily Mail*, Susan Bewley added, 'Quite apart from the possibility of physical addiction, there are strong psychological pressures to stay on HRT. It is supposed to be anti-ageing, so coming off feels like giving up hope of protection from ageing.' Although the researchers stressed that the theory was only a hypothesis, it does have serious implications, not least because of the number of women involved.

Gynaecologist John Studd countered that patients were not addicted to the drug but simply to 'feeling better', and pointed out the benefits of HRT: 'fewer heart attacks, fewer strokes, fewer osteoporotic fractures, less depression, and an extra year or two of life.'

In the meantime the HRT market is growing: in 1992 it is reported to be worth about £40 million. One in ten women over 50 in the UK are reportedly on the treatment, and in parts of the US as many as one in three women. For this reason alone it's vital that we get some real answers to the complex questions surrounding HRT.

The Discreet Charm of HRT

Undoubtedly part both of the allure – and the threat – of HRT lies in its claimed ability to transform. From the first, at least in the popular mind, the drug has straddled that rather fuzzy line between medical treatment and beauty therapy – a 'cosmeceutical' rather than purely a 'pharmaceutical'.

One early advertisement for American gynaecologist Robert A. Wilson's bible *Feminine Forever*, which sold more than 140,000 copies in a year, promised that the book would reveal 'how to avoid menopause completely and stay a romantic, desirable, vibrant woman as long as you live.' In 1989 MP Teresa Gorman – at the same time as saying that the cosmetic question was a side issue – claimed, 'Everyone comments on how rosy my skin is. I can nearly always tell if someone is taking it by the quality of their skin.' An article in the British *Daily Mail* (August 1989) quoted actress Dinah Sheridan, star of *Genevieve* and *The Railway Children*, as saying, 'I'll be 70 next year and I still feel like a middle-aged woman, not a nearly old woman. My quality of life is so good: I feel terrific.' Side issues these may be – but who wouldn't jump at the chance of some HRT in the light of such promises?

Yet, as Dr Val Godfree, deputy director of the Amarant Clinic, set up to promote HRT, admitted in an interview I carried out with her for *She* magazine, 'It's a very personal reaction; some women find it more beneficial than others. I'd never promise that HRT would make a woman look younger. And it doesn't delay ageing. However, a great number of women find that when they regain their self-confidence and esteem, everything else about them improves. Is it the hormones? The truth is we don't know.'

Dr Jean Coope, writing in the doctors' journal *Pulse* (August 1981) posed the question 'Does oestrogen therapy preserve youth and beauty? Our patients in general practice did not think so. Those taking long-term hormone therapy were asked if they or their husbands had noticed an improvement in their appearance. They replied that there was an improvement in the first few weeks but this did not continue.'

One 64-year-old woman, quoted in an issue of *Feeling Good*, the Amarant Trust's own newsletter, spoke for many women when she said, 'As for other improvements people talk about, well to be honest I think it's psychological. I know I'm on HRT and I'm told it works as a sort of pick-me-up, and I leave it at that. I can not see much difference really.'

The idea of taking a drug that will miraculously transform us (or even enable us to stay the same, not getting any older) is enormously attractive. At the same time it is frightening – the stuff of fairy tales rather than of the real world. This perhaps lies at the root of some of the fear that the treatment is 'unnatural'. Youth and beauty *are* prized in our society, as a glance through any women's magazine will reveal. Who wants to find on looking in the mirror that, like the Wicked Stepmother, she is no longer the fairest of all? Yet it is also unrealistic to expect a drug to deliver such attributes. And, as has been pointed out, many of the actresses and film stars on HRT were beautiful to begin with: they didn't get their beauty from implants or patches.

What all the sound and fury surrounding HRT does demonstrate is a real unmet need, on both a physical and emotional level. There is abundant evidence that women undergoing the menopause still aren't getting the support and understanding they deserve. When Teresa Gorman announced that HRT had made a new woman of her, 10,000 women wrote to tell her about the miseries they were undergoing. It was this response that led to the formation of the Amarant Trust, with the aim of raising money to research into the benefits of HRT, and also to the setting up of the Amarant Clinic, where women could get advice and treatment for menopausal symptoms.

Many critics of HRT decry menopause clinics for being little more than HRT-dispensing factories. And it is true that most women do come away clutching a prescription for the drug. However, the fact is that many of those who find their way there are listened to and taken seriously for the first time. A first appointment at the Amarant Clinic, for example, lasts 40 minutes, compared with the average 10 minutes doctors spend with their patients.

Like all complex subjects, HRT *is* controversial. We still don't know how many women would benefit from it if they were on it. And, while we now have a broad general knowledge about some of the risks and benefits, there still remain many unanswered questions.

For example, what effect do the progestogens in HRT have on breast cancer? What doses of the hormones create the best results? Do the newer HRT formulations increase heart disease and stroke or not? Are newer methods of delivering the hormones more or less effective?

In the meantime, each and every one of us has to make up her own mind on the basis of the facts available and on her own personal medical history and needs. Without the skills of unravelling statistics, each and every one of us has to draw up her own personal risk-benefit analysis.

The decision to take HRT will also be based on your attitudes and values, combined with your life experience. If, for example, you have witnessed your mother or a close friend die from breast cancer, your decision may well be very different from someone who has seen a close female relative suffer the agonies of osteoporosis or die of a heart attack. If you are the sort of person who sees no harm in taking a painkiller when you have a headache, your attitude towards taking a drug to combat the unpleasant symptoms of the menopause is likely to be different from a woman who prides herself on getting by without resort to pills and potions, or who prefers to use natural remedies.

In the rest of this book I attempt to clarify some of the issues. But first, what *is* the menopause, and how can HRT help?

CHAPTER ONE

What Is the Menopause?

Alicia was just 23. About to sit nursing finals and busily planning a Christmas wedding, she began experiencing hot flushes, dizziness and aching joints – the classic menopause symptoms.

Her doctor put down her lack of periods to having just come off the Pill, and her other symptoms down to anxiety about the wedding and exams. But after she got married the symptoms continued, the hot flushes becoming even worse.

'I scoured the medical textbooks, convinced I must have something terrible. But menopause was the last thing I thought to look under. I began to think I was going mad.'

Alicia's doctor didn't take her complaints seriously, but eventually agreed to send her to a local gynaecologist, who referred her to one of the leading endocrinologists. Hormone tests and an ultrasound scan revealed that Alicia's ovaries were completely shrivelled. At the age of 24 she had passed through the change of life.

Jane's periods stopped at the age of 36. Within a year she was a virtual invalid. 'I had suffered from backache all my life, but once my periods stopped they became excruciating, and the rest of my bones ached, too. It became so painful to move my arms I had to take time off work; I couldn't walk, I could barely stand without help. And, most frightening of all, I shrank three inches from 5 ft 11 to 5 ft 8.

'The specialist at my local hospital diagnosed osteoporosis and referred me to a gynaecologist who specializes in HRT. By the time I got to see him I was like a rubber doll.'

Jane was prescribed HRT implants. 'Within a month I began to feel more my old self, and within a year I was back to normal and able to return to my job.'

She says: 'I have never felt better. Without HRT I would be in a wheelchair by now.'

Iris's periods continued as normal until she was 51. 'Just the same as usual, but not as long-lasting and more irregular. Then I missed one period. I didn't have flushes and sweats, but I started to get depressed, which is unusual for me. I also started to get vaginal dryness.' She went on HRT for three years before stopping because of the side-effect of even deeper depression. 'My periods had stopped and the menopausal symptoms returned with a vengeance. I had hot flushes, sweats and vaginal dryness. Then I had the most crashing depression, I didn't know what to do.'

So what is the menopause? When does it happen? How long does it last? And what does it feel like? As these accounts show, there are no simple answers.

Strictly speaking, the term 'menopause' refers to a woman's last period. In practice, most people use the word loosely to refer to the whole process of changing from a fertile woman to one who is no longer able to bear children. Doctors call this the perimenopause – the years around the menopause. They also refer to the post-menopause – when the physical and emotional upheavals of the menopause have passed.

The menopause is as much a part of a woman's normal lifecycle as adolescence. In the past 'the change' was spoken of – if at all – in hushed tones, and the lack of guidelines led many women to approach it with dread. Today many women still approach their menopause in fear and ignorance, as a survey carried out by National Opinion Polls (NOP) and the drug company Ciba-Geigy in April 1992 revealed. Out of 1,017 women aged 45 to 58, a staggering two thirds didn't know the cause of the menopause. If you enter the menopause with a positive attitude based on a sound knowledge of what is going on inside your body, you are more likely to be able to cope. If all you know about the menopause is based on half-truths and myths, it's no wonder that you will approach the experience with fear and dread.

What to Expect

In some cases, the periods stop without warning. But usually the first sign that you are approaching the menopause is that your periods become irregular. At first they may come more frequently – every 21 to 24 days as opposed to the usual 28. At this point the amount of blood lost is about the same as usual. Gradually, as the ovaries begin to stop functioning, there tend to be longer intervals in between and you may skip several months altogether. At the same time, the bleeding becomes scantier. However, as the number of cycles without an egg being produced becomes greater, your periods become even more irregular, coming anything from 14 days to several months apart and lasting from a few hours to a few days, with sometimes heavy bleeding.

The average age for the periods to stop is 50 (though smokers, on average, stop a couple of years earlier than this). But a woman's age at menopause can vary enormously. Each woman has her own pattern of development throughout the reproductive years, and just as some girls are fully mature at 13 and others not until their late teens, some women complete the change of life within a year, while for others it may take five years or more.

Some women experience a premature menopause, in their 20s, 30s or early 40s, either because their ovaries fail for some unexplained reason or because of medical treatment which has stopped ovarian function, such as treatment for childhood leukaemia, for example, or a hysterectomy. At the other end of the spectrum, some women don't wave goodbye to their periods until as late as 58 or 59. But for most women 'the change' begins between around 46 and 48 and lasts an average of two to three years.

Cyclical Moves

To understand what happens at the menopause it's necessary to know what happens during the normal menstrual cycle. Every month during the fertile years the body prepares for pregnancy by releasing an egg from the ovaries. If the egg is not fertilized it, together with the lining of the womb which has been preparing for a possible pregnancy, is shed as a period. The whole process is governed by a complex series of hormonal triggers. The ovaries are stimulated into action each month by hormones called gonadotrophins secreted by the pituitary gland. When this happens, between ten and twenty minute follicles begin to ripen on the ovaries. As these follicles ripen they release the hormone oestrogen, which literally means 'egg-making'.

The oestrogen released into the bloodstream sends a chemical message to the hypothalmus (the master gland), which in turn instructs the pituitary to release another gonadotrophin called follicle-stimulating hormone (FSH), which prevents the ovaries from making too much oestrogen.

One of the follicles which is ripening develops more rapidly than the others, and this causes the oestrogen in the bloodstream to peak. This in turn triggers the release of another gonadotrophin from the pituitary called luteinizing hormone (LH), which makes the follicle burst, releasing the egg. This

Patterns of Bleeding

The key feature of the menstrual cycle in the years just before the menopause is that it becomes unsettled and unpredictable. This can make it difficult to distinguish 'normal' from 'abnormal' bleeding. The most usual patterns are:

- More frequent light periods
- Longer intervals between periods
- A gradual decrease in the amount of blood lost
- Occasional missed periods
- Occasional heavy periods
- Irregular periods for a few months, followed by a few months of regular ones
- Regular periods that stop suddenly

Less usual patterns are as follows. If you experience any of these symptoms, it's a good idea to see your doctor:

- Very frequent heavy periods
- Longer periods
- Passing clots
- Bleeding in between periods
- Bleeding which occurs after 12 months free from periods

occurs around the middle of the menstrual cycle.

Meanwhile, back in the ovary, LH encourages the production of the other hormone, progesterone, which means 'pregnancy-making'. It is this hormone that prepares the body to receive the fertilized egg. It thickens the lining of the womb and acts on the breasts, preparing them eventually to make milk. It also works on the adrenal glands, altering the level of fluids and minerals in the body in preparation for a possible pregnancy.

If the egg is not fertilized the ovary stops making progesterone, and as a result of the fall in progesterone levels, the lining of the uterus peels away and is shed with the egg as a period.

Changing Cycles

As menopause approaches, the ovaries begin to become less responsive to the surges of stimulating gonadotrophins from the pituitary. At first the pituitary, failing to get the message from oestrogen levels in the bloodstream, attempts to kick the flagging ovaries into action by sending out another surge of FSH. The ovaries in turn respond but go into uneven action, producing too much oestrogen, so that you may have a sudden, unexpectedly heavy period. The highest levels of gonadotrophins (FSH and LH) are to be found in the two to three years following your last period, as the pituitary strives to drive the failing ovaries.

As a result of these internal changes at first you may notice your periods come more often, as a result of a shortening of the egg development phase of your cycle, due to the unresponsive ovaries. At this stage eggs are still being produced. But as time goes on, the ovaries' continuing lack of response combined with the supply of eggs running out results in waning oestrogen levels. As this happens the length of time between periods tends to lengthen again and sometimes months are skipped altogether. As egg production becomes less and less frequent (the medical term is *anovulatory*), the ovaries stop producing progesterone, too. Eventually oestrogen production falls below a critical level, the lining of the uterus is no longer prepared for pregnancy, and your periods stop altogether.

It is these hormonal fluctuations and the sudden drop in oestrogen levels that produce symptoms such as hot flushes, night sweats and so on which we associate with the change of life.

HRT is meant to 'top up' the body's oestrogen levels and

return them to 'normal' – i.e. what they were before the menopause. One reason for all the controversy surrounding HRT is that after the menopause the body has its own mechanisms for replacing the hormones no longer being produced by the ovaries.

The adrenal glands, which lie above the kidneys, produce a hormone called androstenedione which is capable of being converted by chemical changes in the body into a type of oestrogen. This conversion takes place in fatty tissue. The tendency for women to put on weight after the menopause is sometimes said to be Nature's way of attempting to top up hormonal levels. In some women the oestrogen so manufactured is enough to prevent uncomfortable menopausal symptoms. This may be why overweight women are said to suffer less than slim ones from symptoms such as hot flushes, sweats and osteoporosis.

More controversial is the role of the ovaries themselves. Some experts say that the ovaries make little contribution to hormone levels once the periods have stopped. Others, however, argue that the small but significant amounts of the androgen hormones – androstenedione and testosterone, both of which are able to be converted into oestrogen in the body – secreted by the ovaries can contribute to post-menopausal well-being, once the body has adjusted to lower levels of oestrogen.

In men these same androgen hormones, produced by the testes, are responsible for male characteristics such as facial hair, a deep voice and increased muscle bulk. However, androgens produced by the adrenal glands are less active than the testicular ones, and in any case are converted, in women, into oestrogen. One interesting suggestion is that it is this shift in the balance between oestrogens and androgens that may lie behind the changes in fat metabolism within the bloodstream which bump up women's risk of heart disease after the menopause.

Menopausal Effects

The effects of the menopause can be divided into three main categories: vasomotor, musculo-skeletal and atrophic, and psychological.

VASOMOTOR EFFECTS

Vasomotor effects include hot flushes, sweats, palpitations, headaches and all the symptoms to do with the behaviour of the blood vessels ('vaso' means blood vessels, 'motor' means movement), and the lack of sleep caused by such symptoms.

Hot flushes and night sweats are the most common symptoms of the menopause – about three quarters of women experience them. Yet, amazingly, no one knows exactly why they occur. Curiously, flushes and sweats are not related to the absolute concentration of oestrogen in the bloodstream: neither men nor little girls, who both have low oestrogen levels, suffer flushes, and there is no difference in oestrogen levels in women who suffer flushes and those who don't.

The experts think that they may be caused by the effect of lower levels of oestrogen on receptors in the central nervous system. It is also surmised that for each of us there is an oestrogen level band within which flushes occur. This could explain why eventually the flushes ease off, as oestrogen levels fall below the critical band. Other surmises are that the body eventually adjusts to lower oestrogen levels.

How It Feels

Whatever the cause of these vasomotor effects, the result is a sudden intense sensation of heat and reddening of the upper chest, arms, neck and face. At the same time you may break out into a sweat. Palpitations, dizziness and even fainting can accompany a flush in extreme cases. The flushes can last from several seconds to several minutes and can happen from four or five times a day to several times within an hour. When they occur at night you may wake up so hot and drenched in sweat that you have to change the bedclothes.

'They start in the chest and work their way up to your head and neck until you feel as if you are on fire. Afterwards you feel cold and shivery.'

AMANDA, 32

'It feels as though someone has lit a candle deep inside you and is fanning the flames until they are raging through your entire body.'

EMILY, 52

Doctors classify these vasomotor effects as 'acute symptoms' i.e. they come on suddenly and usually only last for a short time. Most women suffer for from two to five years, though a few unlucky women have symptoms that drag on indefinitely. They tend to happen early on in the menopause, and may even happen before you stop your periods, albeit infrequently.

It's estimated that for two thirds of the women who suffer them, hot flushes and sweats are little more than a minor nuisance. A third of women suffer severely. Women who have had a surgical menopause (a hysterectomy) causing an abrupt stopping of periods are particularly likely to suffer badly, probably because the body finds it difficult to adjust to the sudden drop in oestrogen. A lucky quarter of women sail through the change of life without a single flush. Quite why is one of the great mysteries surrounding the menopause.

Triggers
Flushes aren't harmful, but they can be embarrassing, and this can result in a loss of confidence and self-esteem. One thing to bear in mind is that the more you worry about them the worse they are likely to be. Although you may feel that you are about to burst into flames, most people around you observe little more than a slight pink glow. Anxiety is a known trigger, as are hot weather, moving from a cool to a warm environment, hot, spicy foods, hot drinks and alcohol.

MUSCULO-SKELETAL AND ATROPHIC EFFECTS

These are the changes in tissues and organs such as the skin, the genital tract and the muscles. They include the thinning and drying (*atrophy*, to use the medical term) of the skin both on the body and in the vagina, the latter resulting in dryness, pain and soreness on intercourse and an increase in vaginal infections; urinary infections such as cystitis; flabby breasts; thinning hair; loss of muscular tone leading to prolapse and problems such as stress incontinence (leaking urine when you exert yourself), weight gain, abdominal swelling, and aches and pains in the muscles and joints.

Drs Val Godfree and Malcolm Whitehead, in their book *Hormone Replacement Therapy* (aimed at doctors), describe these effects as 'intermediate' – they are not self-limiting and more women tend to complain of them as time goes on.

> 'My hair and skin were dry and lifeless. We only made love once a month and then with reluctance on my part, I was so dry.'
>
> JULIA, 54

Drs Godfree and Whitehead attribute these symptoms to a lack of oestrogen, which causes drying and thinning of the skin, together with a loss of collagen (a sort of cellular glue that plumps out the cells) from connective tissue, causing joint and muscle aches and pains. Other doctors, however, still question whether these are directly attributable to the effects of waning hormones or are just the natural process of ageing that occurs in both men and women.

PSYCHOLOGICAL EFFECTS

These include a depressing catalogue of effects, listed in one survey as tension, depression, irritability, mood swings, sleep problems, fatigue, lethargy, loss of energy, loss of confidence, inability to concentrate and loss of interest in sex!

'I had a hysterectomy at 44. By 46 I felt dizzy, tired, headachey, tired and listless. The hot sweats were unbearable, every few minutes day and night. I was suicidal. I didn't want to go out.'

JEAN, 50

'I had terrific depression and mood swings, I felt murderous towards my poor darling husband and used to weep like a teenager. I lost my memory. I remember once leaving for work and setting off in the totally opposite direction!'

LIZ, 48

'I became so ill I couldn't go to work, I had to lie down when shopping in town because I got so dizzy. I woke up seven times a night sweating. I couldn't remember things – there were big blanks. I fluffed one very important interview for promotion. I just got into the room and couldn't remember what I wanted to say.'

HANNAH, 51

The question of whether the lack of oestrogen itself causes these problems or whether they are side-effects of physical problems or a result of lifestyle and family pressures that exist at the time, is a moot one. Although it's been estimated that between a quarter and a half of women complain of emotional problems during the menopause, the experts still can't agree why, nor why between half and three-quarters of women don't complain of problems. Are they not reporting them? Are they having them but coping with them? Or are they problem-free?

PHYSICAL CONCERNS
One school of thought argues the physical effects of the menopause are to blame for the emotional ones. Take the vasomotor disturbances for example: flushes and sweats lead to

lack of sleep and tiredness, which in turn lead on to feelings of irritability, mood swings, indecisiveness and lack of concentration. Similarly, loss of interest in sex can be attributed to the pain or soreness when making love caused by vaginal dryness, and an increase in vaginal infections – enough to put anyone off. According to this school of thought, if you can control the physical symptoms the emotional ones will sort themselves out.

HORMONAL UPS AND DOWNS

Another group of experts has it that lack of oestrogen is directly responsible for depression and other psychological symptoms. Gynaecologist John Studd, for example, who treats women privately in Harley Street as well as in clinics at NHS hospitals, is convinced that lack of oestrogen can cause depression. He angered psychiatrists by writing that menopausal women would do better to go on HRT than anti-depressants.

SOCIAL AND EMOTIONAL UPHEAVALS

Yet another theory is that, although hormones do affect the psyche, they have to be seen against a social and emotional backdrop. As Dr Norma Williams and journalist Hetty Einzig wrote in *The New Guide to Women's Health*, 'Hormonal changes can have an effect on the emotions but the pressures a woman experiences in her job and family at this time play a much bigger role in psychological problems. The menopause will not change a happy, secure woman into a miserable, distraught creature – but it could be the last straw for a woman who has been hanging precariously on to her emotional equilibrium for many years.'

I'll be looking at this question in Chapter 4. In the meantime, how can HRT help treat the effects of the menopause?

CHAPTER TWO

How Can HRT Help?

'My doctor wouldn't agree to put me on HRT, she said it was dangerous.'

LINDA, 47

'I went to see my doctor, who said I was too young for HRT. In the end he gave me a drug which was supposed to stop sweats, but it didn't.'

ELLA, 48

'I get cross because doctors are still reluctant to prescribe HRT. My own doctor waved the cancer shroud.'

DIANE, 52

'I heard of HRT 15 years ago and tried to get it from my doctor, who gave it me for 18 months. When I went back for more I saw another partner, who said "No".'

DORIS, 62

In the past, women going to their doctors complaining of menopausal symptoms were met with a shrug and, 'You'll have to get on with it, it's your age.' Today a woman visiting her doctor may still be met with a yawn, but it is also likely that she will be offered a prescription for HRT. Both responses can rouse anger and accusations of disinterest and lack of understanding. But is this really fair?

The fact is, although many of the symptoms of the menopause can be laid at the door of fluctuating oestrogen levels – it's hard to prove they are. Even in the case of hot flushes and night sweats, there's no simple link between low oestrogen levels and experience of symptoms. As to the other host of symptoms, there's *no* universal agreement as to whether they are caused by oestrogen deficiency, nor how far they are helped by it.

The reasoning that goes 'if women experience symptoms during the menopause, it must be because of a shortage of hormones; therefore if you give back the hormones all will be well,' is seductively simple. It's also argued that because you are merely putting back what is missing, it isn't unnatural or harmful. However, as Dr Andrew Dunford, a medical doctor who is also a herbalist, points out, 'I can't help feeling that if the hormones run out they do so for a reason.' And even Drs Godfree and Whitehead, unabashed enthusiasts of HRT, admit in their book *HRT: Your Questions Answered*: 'Post-menopausal women are highly placebo-responsive.' In other words, some women will get better *no matter what treatment you give them.*

The question then arises: should such women be given HRT, which may have potentially harmful side-effects, or should they be given something simpler that has no side-effects? What we need are more and better controlled trials both of HRT and the alternatives, combined with better support and understanding for women undergoing the change of life.

The Facts About HRT

HRT consists of low doses of the hormone oestrogen. It is designed to replace the body's own natural supply of oestrogen, which diminishes as the ovaries cease working. It also contains (for women who haven't had a hysterectomy) the other female sex hormone, progesterone.

HRT is often spoken of as if it were a single drug. In fact it comes in many different forms and strengths. This means there are literally hundreds of combinations, and one of them might be right for you. The skill of the doctor lies in tailoring the treatment to your individual needs. If you aren't happy with what you have been prescribed, go back and ask to try something else. In this chapter I outline the different types of HRT, to enable you to understand what might be prescribed for you, and to help you make informed choices about what might be the best regime for you.

OESTROGEN
There are several different forms of the hormone oestrogen in the body, and two types of oestrogen used in HRT: natural and synthetic.

Natural Oestrogen
The natural oestrogen used in HRT isn't extracted from humans as you might expect. This most common form, conjugated equine oestrogen, actually comes from the urine of pregnant mares. Other types of natural oestrogen are synthesized in the laboratory; yet they are called 'natural' because their action in the bloodstream is similar to that of the oestrogen produced by the ovaries before the menopause.

Synthetic Oestrogen
This, on the other hand, is different in chemical structure to the type of oestrogen produced by the ovary. This is the sort of oestrogen used in the Pill. In order to stop ovulation this sort is much more powerful than the natural oestrogens used in HRT. It is not used in HRT because it raises oestrogen levels in the blood to too high a level, and may also be capable of altering the levels of certain harmful blood factors in the liver, which raises the risk of blood clots.

PROGESTOGEN

Because oestrogen alone can heighten the risk of endometrial cancer in women who have not had a hysterectomy, another hormone, progestogen is prescribed in pill form for the last ten to twelve days of the cycle.

Progestogen is a synthetic version of the female sex hormone, progesterone. Remember, synthetic means it isn't similar in structure to the natural hormone produced by the ovary.

In fact, there are two sorts of progestogens. Firstly there is a sort (called C 21s) whose chemical structure is related to progesterone itself. Secondly there is the sort (called C 19s) that is structurally related to the male sex hormone, testosterone. Natural progesterone is not suitable for use in HRT, because in order to protect the womb it has to be given in two large daily doses. Natural progesterone given in doses this high could produce unwelcome side-effects, such as drowsiness. If for any reason you can't tolerate synthetic progestogens, you may be prescribed natural progesterone in suppository form. The drawback of drowsiness can be minimized by inserting the suppository last thing at night.

The progestogen element in HRT causes a light bleeding once a month. The bleeding helps slough off the lining of the womb. If there is no bleeding it simply means there is no womb lining being formed.

Nowadays doctors tend to favour prescribing oestrogen continuously, with progestogen added for 12 days of the cycle. This avoids problems of breakthrough bleeding and the return of severe menopausal symptoms. It's also thought to lower the risk of endometrial cancer. If you start taking HRT while you are still having periods, the progestogen part of the dose will be timed to produce bleeding at the same time as your natural period.

Continuous Combined Therapy

Some doctors now prescribe a continuous combined therapy, in which oestrogen and progestogen are both taken every day. This avoids the inconvenience of a monthly bleed.

As yet there is no long-term information on the effects of this continuous combined form of treatment, and it's not yet known whether it has any adverse effects on the womb lining. For this reason you'll be advised to have a sample of womb lining tested every 12 to 18 months. This is done using a simple suction device, which avoids the need for a conventional D & C under general anaesthetic. The procedure takes about 15 minutes.

Types of HRT

There are different ways of taking HRT: orally as pills, as a vaginal cream or pessary, a skin patch, or an implant. There are also different dosages of both oestrogen and progestogen. Different doctors tend to have their own favourite methods, but providing there are no medical reasons why you shouldn't have a particular regime, it's up to you to decide. The aim is to produce a similar balance of hormones to that which existed before the menopause. Each of the four main types of HRT has its advantages and disadvantages. The type you end up with will depend on what your doctor thinks would suit you best and the method you would prefer.

PILLS
These are the most common form of HRT in the UK, US and Australia and there are several different brands available. Unless you have had a hysterectomy, you will be prescribed a combination of oestrogen and progestogen, which come in a

three- or, more usually, four-week calendar pack, similar to those used for the Pill. Sometimes the tablets are colour coded, so you know when you are taking oestrogen, when progestogen, and when a combination of the two.

Sometimes the oestrogen and progestogen are combined in one tablet. These combinations don't offer as much flexibility as individually prescribed oestrogen and progestogen, however they are convenient to use.

Advantages
They are easy to take and the dose can be easily adjusted.

Disadvantages
They may cause indigestion. If you are a disorganized type you may forget to take them. May cause irregular bleeding, especially if you have only recently had your last period.

CREAMS AND PESSARIES
These are usually prescribed if your main problem is a dry vagina or urethra. You apply them directly into the vagina with a special applicator. They will not stain the bedclothes.

Advantages
They are easy to use. If you don't like the idea of taking HRT in pill form, or if your only symptom is vaginal dryness, they provide relief with just the minimum dose of oestrogen.

Disadvantages
They don't offer protection against osteoporosis or heart disease, and don't usually stop hot flushes. They may also be absorbed by your partner and cause him to feel unwell! – The answer is not to insert the cream or suppositories immediately before making love.

PATCHES
These are small transparent sticky 'plasters' containing oestrogen, which are applied to the skin of the lower abdomen

and changed every three to four days. The oestrogen is absorbed into the skin. If you still have your womb you will need to take progestogen tablets as well for 12 days of the cycle.

Advantages
Oestrogen taken in this way doesn't pass through the liver, so the risks of side-effects are lowered. For this reason many doctors prefer this method. Patches are also said to provide a more constant level of oestrogen.

Disadvantages
The patch may need to be moved to a different spot twice a week, and more often in hot weather, to avoid skin irritation. They can come off in the bath or when you go swimming. If sunbathing, you won't tan where the patch is.

IMPLANTS
Tiny pellets of oestrogen about the size of an apple pip are inserted under the skin of the abdomen or buttock. These pellets then release oestrogen gradually into the bloodstream. The effects last about six months. Unless you have had a hysterectomy, you will have to take progestogen tablets as well for around 12 days a month.

Advantages
You don't have to remember to take tablets. Avoids the disadvantages of patches, while still not passing through the liver.

Disadvantages
The dose cannot be modified once you have had the implant inserted. Removal is difficult. There is also the possible danger of addiction (see page 84).

NEW TREATMENTS

Tibolone

This product, which goes under the brand name *Livial*, is a synthetic hormone. It has the properties of an oestrogen, a progestogen and an androgen (the hormones produced by the testes in men and the adrenal glands in both sexes). It seems to control menopausal symptoms without producing the withdrawal bleeding that some women find such a nuisance. However, the drug is as yet too new for any long-term risks to be known about. And it's not yet known whether it has a similar protective value as conventional HRT against bone or heart disease.

Testosterone

Some doctors are now using implants of the male sex hormone testosterone, which is capable of being converted in the body into oestrogen. Women make small amounts of this hormone, which is said to add to the beneficial effects of HRT when given in small doses.

However, this treatment is extremely controversial. Its only proven effect is its capacity to boost waning sexual desire. However, some women also report relief of tiredness and lethargy, especially those who have had their ovaries removed as part of a hysterectomy.

The Case for HRT

There is undoubted evidence that HRT can alleviate many of the symptoms of the menopause. The definite benefits include relief from hot flushes and vaginal dryness. The benefits yet to be proved conclusively, include relief from cystitis, depression, the 'jotter syndrome', carpal tunnel syndrome, and dry skin and hair.

RELIEF FROM HOT FLUSHES

Studies have shown time and time again that oestrogen can help with the vasomotor symptoms, such as flushing, sweating and insomnia. Studies have shown a dramatic decrease in flushing, with some women reporting complete relief in just a few days, and the majority within three months.

> 'Three weeks after being put on HRT I didn't have a single symptom.'
>
> EMILY, 52

Others find HRT doesn't always quell symptoms completely: a sudden hot spell, a long course of antibiotics (which can interfere with oestrogen metabolism) and stress at work or home can bring on an attack. Going off HRT suddenly can also lead to a rebound in symptoms, which is why doctors advise tailing off doses gradually over several weeks or months (see page 56).

Is It for Me?

If flushes are making your life thoroughly miserable, there are no reasons why you shouldn't have HRT (see page 93), and you feel it might be for you, it could well be worth giving it a try.

RELIEF FROM VAGINAL DRYNESS

This is slightly more complicated. Reliable studies have shown that oestrogen is effective in treating vaginal dryness and restoring comfort when making love, so increasing desire and satisfaction. The dose of oestrogen needed to treat vaginal changes is less than is needed for treating flushes, and, as mentioned earlier, it can be prescribed as a cream.

On the other hand, there is some evidence that the combined form of HRT (that includes progesterone) counteracts some of these beneficial effects. More controversial still, some doctors also prescribe an implant of the male hormone testosterone to boost desire, in spite of the fact that studies have failed to show conclusively that this is any better than giving oestrogen on its own.

The whole question is complicated because, as has been said many times, the brain is the biggest sex organ. Physically, the more you make love the better shape your vagina will be in. But there are all sorts of emotional and mental reasons that may lie behind a reluctance to make love or taking longer to get aroused. These factors, as well as the physical ones, need to be tackled.

If vaginal dryness is your only troublesome symptom and you don't like the idea of taking HRT, there are other lubricating jellies and creams available. *KY Jelly* is the most tried and tested. A newer product, *Replens*, works by holding the skin's own natural moisture in the vagina (rather like wallpaper paste holds water in suspension!). It is odourless and not greasy at all, and has to be applied every three days. Many women prefer it to having to mess about with creams or jellies when they want to make love.

Is It for Me?
If you have reason to believe lack of lubrication and thinning skin is the main reason why you no longer enjoy lovemaking, and there are no contraindications, again it could be worth giving HRT a try.

RELIEF FROM CYSTITIS
Some women find that they suffer from cystitis-like symptoms after the menopause – needing to run to the loo more often than usual, having to get up at night to pass water, and discomfort or pain on urinating. Yet when tests are carried out, no signs of urinary infection are discovered. Some studies have shown that HRT clears symptoms up within just a couple of weeks of treatment.

This is not the whole story, however. Although urinary symptoms are common complaints among women attending hospital menopause clinics, some studies have shown no difference between women's symptoms before and after the menopause. This finding would suggest that a shortage of oestrogen isn't the cause. Furthermore, it could be that when women suffering flushes and sweats are given oestrogen they sleep better, and so don't need to get up during the night.

RELIEF FROM DEPRESSION

'Within a month I'd stopped having sweats with the result that I sleep better, I've got a new interest in life. We had become bowlers but I had got to stage of getting so tired I couldn't do it. I still don't want to go in pubs or crowds, though.'

JILL, 53

'In my job you have to be presentable and not forget what you are saying half way through. HRT made me feel better and gave me back my self-esteem.'

EMMA, 54

Oestrogen certainly seems to have a pharmacological effect on mood. Furthermore, by helping with the physical symptoms, it can result in increased energy and a consequent boost in self-confidence and self-esteem – both important factors in mental well-being. On the other hand there is the danger that, like any other anti-depressive drug, HRT merely masks symptoms of depression rather than encouraging women to make the life changes that might lead to them feeling better.

RELIEF FROM THE 'JOTTER SYNDROME'

This is the name given by doctors to the poor concentration and memory some women complain of: the condition becomes so bad that women have to make lists to enable them to remember what they have to do. Lack of concentration is a known feature of depression (see above). Again the question is whether the symptom is due to oestrogen deficiency or to other stresses that coincide with the menopause.

Many women do report an improvement in memory after beginning treatment, however. Whether this is purely to do with oestrogen or again to relief from physical symptoms is again debatable.

For a fuller discussion of HRT's beneficial (or otherwise) effects on emotional symptoms of the menopause, see Chapter 4.

RELIEF FROM CARPAL TUNNEL SYNDROME

Carpal tunnel syndrome is a numbness, tingling and pain in the thumb, index and middle fingers. It is often worse at night. The condition can affect one or both hands and can cause weakness of the thumb. It's caused by pressure on the nerve that runs from the wrist into the hands via a gap called the 'carpal tunnel'. The condition occurs most often in pregnant women, middle-aged women, and in women who have just gone on the pill – all of which suggests there may be a hormone connection. Traditionally treatment consists of rest, injections of steroid drugs or surgery to relieve pressure on the nerve. However, recent research has shown that the syndrome can be relieved by HRT.

RELIEF FROM DRY SKIN AND HAIR

'I felt my life was cut off dramatically at an early stage. HRT takes me back 20 years, the energy is enormous. My hair is bouncy and shiny. I'd put on three stone in weight, but since the HRT I've successfully dieted – before it was too much effort.'

LOUISE, 49

Even more open to question are the cosmetic effects of oestrogen on hair and skin. The skin and hair do tend to become dryer and less elastic as we get older, but are these natural features of ageing or are they symptoms of oestrogen deficiency which can be improved by HRT? Enthusiasts of HRT claim that oestrogen boosts the rate of collagen production – the cellular glue that plumps out skin and hair, restoring their thickness and elasticity.

What's more, although some women experience improvements in skin and hair texture, HRT can't delay the

development of wrinkles. These are a result of photoageing –
years of exposure to the sun and the elements.

And while some women claim they notice an improvement
in the texture of their hair while on HRT, it can't stop hair loss,
which is again a result of ageing rather than lack of hormones.
Even if HRT has these beneficial effects on hair and skin, you
may question whether it's a good idea to take powerful drugs
with as yet unknown long-term effects simply for their cosmetic
benefits.

So far of course I haven't mentioned two of the major long-
term health benefits of taking HRT: the alleged prevention of
heart disease and osteoporosis. These are so important in terms
of our future health and well-being, and the issues surrounding
them are so complex, that the whole of the next chapter is
devoted to them.

Possible Side-effects of HRT

Some women feel dramatically better on HRT. Others suffer
from various physical and emotional side-effects and stop the
treatment.

Some risks and side-effects are dependent on the way the
therapy is taken. A survey carried out by *Woman's Realm*
magazine in association with the drug company Schering (1992)
discovered that many women go off HRT because of initial side-
effects that could have been eliminated by changing the dose or
type of therapy. Bear this in mind, and remember you may need
to have your treatment adjusted several times before you get it
right.

Side-effects are often the body's response to treatment, and
disappear within three months. Many of them are related
to the progestogen part of the treatment, which can cause
Premenstrual Syndrome (PMS)-type symptoms. You may be
especially vulnerable if you previously suffered from PMS while
you were still menstruating.

Many of the side-effects go away of their own accord. For example, breast tenderness – a common problem – usually disappears within six to eight weeks. Indigestion and nausea may also be a problem when you first start to take the treatment. It usually disappears, though around two in fifty women on the pill type of HRT and one in fifty using patches may continue to experience discomfort.

A lot of the side-effects can be alleviated by paying attention to your lifestyle. For example, a diet rich in fruit and vegetables and low in salt can help with problems like fluid retention. Too much caffeine can aggravate breast tenderness. Red wine, chocolate and cheese may trigger headaches in some women. So, maintaining a healthy diet, cutting down on coffee, tea and alcohol, kicking the weed if you smoke and taking regular exercise are all valuable whether or not you go on HRT. Some of the alternative therapies suggested in Chapter 6 may be helpful for coping with side-effects, too.

If the side-effects don't disappear, or if you find them incapacitating, don't suffer in silence. Contact your doctor or practice nurse. A change of dosage can often sort the problems out. If despite trying a change of method or dose the side-effects continue, you will have to decide whether the potential benefits which made you decide to take HRT in the first place are more important to you than the unwelcome effects of the drug.

Don't Forget: Even if you suffer unwelcome side-effects, it's vital to keep taking the progestogen part of the treatment to protect against endometrial cancer.

HRT *and Side-effects*

Possible Side-effects of Natural Oestrogens

- Indigestion and nausea
- Tender breasts
- Leg cramps
- Fluid retention
- Vaginal discharge

Emotional and Physical Side-effects of Progestogens

Emotional

- Aggression
- Irritability
- Anxiety
- Restlessness
- Panic attacks
- Depression
- Mood swings
- Poor concentration
- Forgetfulness
- Lethargy

Physical

- Acne
- Greasy skin
- Abdominal cramps/bloating
- Fluid retention
- Weakness
- Headaches
- Dizziness
- Breast tenderness
- Hot flushes

Getting Advice About HRT

Is Your Doctor Really Listening?

A survey carried out by nurse Joyce Masling and reported in *Nursing Times* (September 1988) showed that 77 per cent of women had heard of HRT, while 23 per cent did not know it existed. Twelve per cent were given the drug by their doctors, 3 per cent were refused it. Masling says, 'The feeling that came across was either that [women] did not know enough about it, or they did not want it, as they were afraid of the side-effects, or they did not realize it was freely available.'

Less than half of the same women's GPs replied to a letter. Just over three quarters said they had time to discuss menopausal problems. However, 22 per cent said they didn't have enough time due to pressure of work, and short length of appointments.

None of the doctors frequently prescribed tranquillizers for menopausal symptoms. However, almost half of the doctors said they occasionally prescribed tranquillizers for menopausal symptoms, and just over half said it was never necessary to refer women to a specialist. Just over half never suggested any alternative source of help and advice.

It is worth remembering that not all doctors are knowledgeable about the various types of HRT. If you aren't satisfied with your treatment and your doctor is unwilling to help, you might be better off attending one of the specialist menopause clinics, which have greater experience of and interest in HRT.

Whether you decide to see your doctor or attend a specialist menopause clinic, there are certain things you can expect.

Visiting a Clinic

It's vital that whoever you see takes the time to talk to you and listen, as well as carrying out the various physical checks. This listening element is just as important as the medical check-ups, especially as all many women need is simple reassurance that they are not alone. Don't allow yourself to be bulldozed into accepting a prescription for HRT if that is not what you want. On the other hand, it's up to you to explain if you don't want HRT, as the doctor may otherwise just assume that that is what you have come for.

BEFORE YOU GO ON HRT

When you first go to your doctor or to a special menopause clinic, the most likely procedure will be:

- Your full medical history and family medical history will be taken. Before you visit the doctor, sit down and make a list of all the illnesses you have suffered in the past. Don't forget to mention any hereditary diseases such as a strong history of breast cancer.
- You will be weighed.
- There will be a breast examination and mammogram if you haven't had one within the last three years.
- You will be given a full physical examination.
- Your blood-pressure will be measured.
- You will be given an internal vaginal examination.
- The doctor will take a cervical smear if you haven't had one within the last three years.
- Your urine will be tested for sugar.
- Sometimes a blood test will be administered to determine your hormone levels.
- Sometimes a bone density scan or biochemical test will be carried out to check your risk of osteoporosis.

CHECKS TO CHECK OUT

If you decide to go on HRT, you will need regular medical

checks. This can be both a bonus or a bore, depending on your attitude. The advantage of having regular check-ups is that potentially severe illnesses such as breast cancer, cervical cancer and so on may be picked up early on. The disadvantage is that your life becomes heavily 'medicalized' and you may find yourself being prescribed unnecessary treatment for minor conditions that might have gone away of their own accord given time, or that could have been treated by relatively simple self-help or alternative methods.

WHEN YOU ARE ON HRT

When you first go on HRT your progress should be carefully monitored. You should then be checked after three months to make sure the treatment suits you and that any side-effects have settled down. After that, follow up appointments will vary from between six months to a year, depending on your doctor's practice.

There should be time at each visit to discuss your treatment and any problems you may be having with it. Don't forget to mention any breakthrough bleeding. This bleeding may simply indicate the need for a change of dose. It could, however, be a sign of something more serious, in which case it may need further investigation such as a D & C to take a sample from the lining of the womb.

At each visit the doctor will check the following:

- your blood-pressure
- your weight.

He or she will also ask you about your bleeding pattern, and you will be given a breast examination and an internal examination.

Possible Extra Tests
- If you have fibroids, a vaginal ultrasound scan may be recommended once a year to check they are not growing.

- Bone density scans may be recommended for some women.

If at any time you develop any of the following symptoms, see the doctor without delay, as they could be signs of serious illness:

- irregular bleeding
- pains in your calves or chest
- sudden shortness of breath
- severe headaches or dizziness
- jaundice
- any unusual change in your breasts such as a lump, dimple or puckering.

How Long Should I Take It?

Some women take HRT for just a few months; others carry on taking it for the rest of their lives. Your decision depends on:

- why you are taking it in the first place
- whether you think the side-effects (such as a return of 'periods') are too much of a nuisance, and
- whether you consider having to make regular visits to the doctor a bind.

If you are taking HRT because you had a premature menopause, then long-term treatment is more likely to be recommended.

If you are taking it to quell flushes and sweats you might consider taking it for up to two years, after which time the flushes will usually have resolved themselves.

If you are taking HRT to prevent osteoporosis, then you need to take it for at least five years (most doctors would recommend taking it for 10 to 15 years). Protection from heart disease may take two to three years, but HRT is said to be just as effective on this front whether you begin in your 50s or your 70s.

However, some studies have shown some of the protective effects to be lost within two years of stopping therapy.

Stopping Treatment

When you come off HRT you should do so gradually, over the course of two or three months under supervision of your doctor. If you come off suddenly, this may trigger a sudden return of unpleasant symptoms. The oestrogen dose can be slowly tailed off. You may find you experience a temporary return of flushes, sweats and emotional problems, but these aren't usually serious and will wear off as you gradually stop taking the treatment. Some doctors advise you to continue to take progestogen until you finish treatment, to avoid build-up of the womb lining. However, not all doctors believe this is necessary. Once you do stop progestogen, of course, your 'period' will become much lighter or it may stop altogether. You might also experience a light withdrawal bleed of two to three days' length when you stop HRT altogether.

CHAPTER THREE

HRT: *Protection against Bone and Heart Disease?*

One of the most powerful arguments in favour of HRT is the protection it is said to confer against two major threats to health and well-being as we get older: osteoporosis (the brittle bone disease) and heart disease. However, as always with the HRT story, the arguments are far from simple.

Calcium and Your Bones

We can probably all remember as children seeing little old ladies with humped backs and walking sticks. In those days we didn't know why they were so fragile. Today we have a label to hang of the symptoms of shrinking, thinning bones – osteoporosis, which means literally 'porous bones'.

We tend to think of our skeleton as an unchanging framework. In fact, bone is living tissue, which throughout our lives is being broken down and reformed in a continuous cycle of loss and renewal. Cells called *osteoclasts* eat away at the bone, releasing calcium into the bloodstream; at the same time, cells called *osteoblasts* fill in the holes, topping up calcium levels in the bone. If the body is short of calcium, because you aren't getting enough in your diet, for example, or are physically inactive, the body attempts to correct this by releasing calcium from the bones into the bloodstream. On the other hand, hard physical exercise or work such as gardening, and a diet rich in calcium, helps calcium to be absorbed from the bloodstream into the bones.

Bone renewal is at its most rapid during childhood and the teenage years because we are growing. So long as we eat a good diet and get enough exercise, until around the age of 30 bone formation and bone reabsorption are pretty evenly balanced. From about the age of 40 we all lose more calcium from the bones, causing them to become brittle and more easily broken. This means that osteoporosis is a natural part of ageing for both men and women.

Although all bones undergo these changes, not all of them are affected in quite the same way. There are two types of bone tissue: cortical bone and trabecular bone. Cortical bone makes up most of the skeleton and is solid and dense; trabecular bone, found in the vertebrae, pelvis and ends of the long bones, has a lattice-like, porous texture. Despite its fragile appearance trabecular bone is enormously strong; nevertheless it is most vulnerable to loss. Women lose about 35 per cent of cortical bone and 50 per cent of trabecular during a lifetime, compared to the approximately 25 and 35 per cent respectively lost by men.

In women the whole process of bone loss speeds up after the menopause, leaving us vulnerable to fractures – particularly in the wrists, hips and vertebra, as well as the ribs and the bone of the upper arm (the humerus), where more trabecular bone is concentrated. By the age of 60 one in four women will have oestoporosis. By the age of 80 two in five have will have sustained a broken bone, and one in eight will have had a fractured hip: one of the most disabling fractures, and a major cause of death.

The facts behind these dismal statistics are these: before the menopause oestrogen helps the bones restore calcium, so helping keep them strong and healthy. We don't know quite how oestrogen does this, but it's known that there are oestrogen receptors on the oestoblasts – the bone-rebuilding cells. At the same time, oestrogen puts a damper on the activity of osteoclasts, the cells that eat away at the bone. In addition, it's thought that oestrogens also act indirectly by stimulating secretion of the hormone calcitonin, which controls levels of calcium in the blood and slows the rate at which calcium is lost.

Following the menopause, loss of bone mass can occur at a frightening rate – but this varies from woman to woman. Once oestrogen levels fall the osteoclasts roar into action at a much faster rate than before, stripping the bones of calcium. At the same time the osteoblasts work more slowly, so that the balance of bone loss and bone manufacture is upset and more bone is lost than made. By the age of 70 a woman can have lost a third of her bone mass. The process is particularly rapid in the first five years after the menopause, when the loss of trabecular bone in the spine can be as much as 5 per cent a year. Fortunately things don't go on at this alarming rate: by eight to ten years after the menopause the degree of bone loss slows down. The problem is that if you haven't much bone mass to begin with and you lose it at a very rapid rate, the bones are so weakened that further loss renders them ever more vulnerable.

What is worrying is that osteoporosis is on the increase – many experts believe because of our modern sedentary lifestyle. Linda Edwards of the National Osteoporosis Society has said, *'Post-menopausal osteoporosis is now the commonest metabolic disease in the West, and so far HRT is the only medical treatment which we know will prevent it.'*

BALANCING THE RISKS

All of us lose oestrogen at the menopause, but not all women suffer osteoporosis. There are three main factors that determine your risk: your peak bone mass at maturity – and although this is partly genetically determined there are lots of things you can do to maximize the strength of your bones – the age at which you start to lose bone and the rate of bone loss once you hit the menopause. HRT can affect the latter two factors, and some promising new research shows that regular weight-bearing exercise and taking calcium supplements can help, too. One piece of good news is that no one has discovered any links between symptoms such as flushes and sweats and osteoporosis. So just because you suffer badly from the early menopausal miseries doesn't necessarily mean you will also suffer from its later effects.

Am I at Risk?

How do you know if you will be one of the one in four women who contracts osteoporosis? You are more at risk if:

- You have had your ovaries removed or put out of action by medical treatment such as radiotherapy, or undergone a premature menopause (before the age of 40–45).

  See Chapter 5. Such women lose bone over a longer period of time, and bone loss is also greater than after a natural menopause.
- You are small-boned and slim.

  Heavier women's bones and muscles have to work harder to carry that extra weight, which helps keep calcium levels in the bones high. And more fat means more oestrogen in the system. The super-slim role-models we are all encouraged to emulate could be at least partly responsible for the growing epidemic of osteoporosis we are now seeing.
- You live a sedentary life.

  Walking, running, dancing and so on – the so-called weight-bearing exercises, stimulate bone growth and calcification. Several recent studies have shown the beneficial effects of even small extra amounts of exercise after the menopause – so leave the car at home and walk!
- You are of Northern European, Asian, Chinese or Japanese origin.

Black women and those of Mediterranean descent are less at risk of osteoporosis. There may be some differences in the hormonal profile of these women, or something in their diets could lead them to have stronger bones in the first place. Women who live in countries with a lot of sunshine tend to be at less risk, too, as vitamin D, which is metabolized from exposure to sunlight, is necessary to create calcium in the body.

- You have a family history of osteoporosis.

The disease tends to run in families, perhaps because of genetic factors which determine bone loss and rate of loss. Shared environment and lifestyle factors may also play a part. For example, children of smokers are far more likely to smoke. A child who takes little exercise and whose diet is low in calcium in childhood can predispose her to the illness.

- You have to take steroid drugs for any medical condition, such as asthma, diabetes, or thyroid problems.

Steroids decrease bone formation and increase bone loss.

- You have been on constant slimming diets or other faddy eating regimes, or have ever been anorexic.

Restricting your diet can leave you short of calcium so that your body has to draw on the calcium stores in the bones. In the case of anorexia, the periods often stop, leading to low levels of oestrogen and a consequent rise in bone loss. We all need 1 gram of calcium a day; after the menopause we need even more – around 1.4 grams a day. Some doctors recommend taking calcium supplements to ensure that we get the necessary amount.

- You eat a lot of meat.

Too much protein in the diet boosts calcium excretion.

- You smoke.

  Smoking cuts oestrogen output and leads on to an earlier menopause. Even passive smokers have been found to have an earlier menopause. Secondly, smoking affects other glands – including the parathyroids, which control blood calcium levels. Finally, smokers tend to be slimmer, exercise less, and have poorer diets than non-smokers.

- You are a heavy drinker.

  Your risk of osteoporosis could be greater if you drink heavily because of the direct toxic effect on the ovaries caused by too much alcohol. Heavy alcohol consumption is also sometimes linked to a lifestyle of poor nutrition, below-average weight, smoking, lack of exercise and liver disease. One study shows that in women in their late 40s consuming more than two alcoholic drinks a day, hip bone density is decreased by 12 per cent – a good reason to go on the wagon, or at least limit your alcohol intake. Heavy drinking can also can also lead to a greater tendency to falls and accidents!

- You drink a lot of tea or coffee.

  Caffeine leaches calcium from the bloodstream.

- You have never had any children.

  For some (as yet unknown) reason, which may be to do with higher oestrogen levels during pregnancy, the more children a woman has had the lower her risk of osteoporosis.

Some doctors go so far as to say that because of the risks of osteoporosis, all of us should take hormones for a few years at the menopause. However, even with a high number of risk factors, some women confound all the predictions.

BONE-DENSITY TESTING

A more accurate measure of whether or not you are likely to suffer osteoporosis is said to be a bone scan. Conventional X-rays can only detect osteoporosis when around 30 per cent of bone has been lost. However a newer, more sophisticated technique of scanning – dual photon absorptiometry – is able to produce rapid, highly accurate results. A scan carried out at age 50 can predict your bone mass at age 70, allowing the doctor to make an estimate of your personal risk. If you have a high bone mass, then even if you lose bone rapidly, your final level will never be as low as women who have a low bone mass to start with. If you have low bone mass at menopause then you may have a high risk of osteoporosis, and whatever your predicted rate of bone loss, you can't afford to lose any more bone. For maximum accuracy, especially for women who fall between the two extremes, several scans are necessary to plot the rate of bone loss, before a final decision can be made about HRT.

Not all experts agree, however, that bone scanning is a reliable way of detecting bone loss. They argue that low bone mass has not been causally linked with an increased risk of fracture in later life, and question the value of routine screening. However, as this is the best method we have at present, it may be worth thinking about if several of the risk factors listed apply to you.

BONE TURNOVER

A second biochemical screening method, which measures concentrations of various chemicals in the blood and the urine, has been developed to show the rate at which bone is lost. Danish researchers showed that combining this test with measurements of height and weight picked up 79 per cent of 'fast bone losers' and 78 per cent of 'slow bone losers'.

The advantage of this simpler method is that it doesn't need any expensive equipment, so it can be done at a doctor's premises. Researchers in another Danish study, reported in the *British Medical Journal* (19 October 1991), suggested that a combination of a baseline measurement of bone mass in the forearm, using a simple type of bone scan called single photon absorptiometry, combined with measuring the various chemicals in the blood and urine (taking a biochemical profile) at the menopause, is the best predictor of those at risk of osteoporosis.

At present none of these tests is widely available, so it's up to you to seek them out if you think you may be at risk of osteoporosis. Many menopause clinics now have bone scanners, or will know where you can go to get a reliable scan. You can also pay to have a bone scan.

As with any medical test, the reliability of the results depends on the experience of the operator, so it's worth searching around to find a clinic that sees a lot of menopausal women. The National Osteoporosis Society (see the Useful Addresses section for the address) will send you a list of hospitals with bone scanners in your area.

TIME FACTORS
Although HRT can halt bone loss any time after the menopause, it's most effective when begun during the accelerated phase of bone loss – that is, during the first few years after your last period. Any sort of HRT seems to work – patches, implants or pills, so long as you get a sufficient dose of oestrogen. *Taking HRT for at least five years can cut your risk of hip fracture by half and your risk of crush fracture of the spine – the most common type of osteoporotic fracture-even more, bringing the risk in line with men of the same age.* But bone experts say that for maximum benefit HRT should be continued for ten to fifteen years. And certainly if you have had a premature menopause, you need to start taking it as soon as your periods stop, and continue taking it until you are 55.

Once you stop taking the treatment, bone loss continues at the rate normally seen at the time of the menopause. Because of this, some doctors even claim that treatment should be continued until the age of 70. One study showed that bone loss speeded up once HRT was discontinued, which led to the conclusion that therapy of between two and four years was useless. However, as the study was carried out on women who had undergone premature menopause, who are known to lose bone more rapidly anyway, it is difficult to draw any firm conclusions.

What isn't so firmly established is whether HRT can do anything to help women who already have osteoporosis. Some studies have shown that oestrogen improves bone density slightly and reduces the risk of fracture. However, other studies have to be weighed against this, as they show that, for HRT to be effective, it should be given close to menopause. It may not be so effective later on. Secondly, women in their 70s may not want to go back to the inevitable 'periods' that accompany HRT.

OTHER OPTIONS

What if you don't want or can't take HRT? Fortunately, new drugs have now been developed to treat osteoporosis, though none so far to prevent it. The first is *calcitonin*, the thyroid hormone which controls calcium levels in the blood. It works by slowing down the rate at which bone is resorbed by the body, by quelling the activity of the osteoclast (bone-eating) cells.

One drawback is that calcitonin has to be given by injection; however, a nasal spray is being developed that should make the drug easier to take. A few women find it causes flushing and nausea. These side-effects usually disappear with time.

Even more promising is a non-hormonal drug called *Didronel* (etidronate disodium), one of a group of chemicals called biphosphonates, originally developed by washing powder companies to try and counteract the effects of hard water! The drug works by inhibiting the reabsorption of bone, which occurs within two weeks of the bone-remodelling cycle. The drug works by sticking to the surface of bone, so it can't be reabsorbed by the bone demolition cells, the osteoclasts. Research published in the *New England Journal of Medicine* (1991) showed that the drug increased bone mass by 5 per cent after three years of treatment and also led to a dramatic reduction in the incidence of spinal fracture. The drugs are taken in pill form for 14 days, followed by a calcium supplement for two and a half months.

The biggest drawback is that the drug is not very well absorbed by mouth, so has to be taken on an empty stomach; some women find it causes minor stomach upsets.

More controversial is the use of calcium supplements. Many doctors claim they are useless, however some studies have shown that supplements containing over 1 gram calcium a day reduce bone reabsorption. Although they don't prevent loss of trabecular bone, they do decrease loss of cortical bone. The problem is we don't know which women would benefit most, nor how much calcium is needed – one study says 1.5 grams, another has shown that as little as 450 mg can be effective – nor whether other lifestyle factors such as smoking, drinking and so on can affect the beneficial effects of calcium supplementation. One interesting study suggested that giving a calcium supplement might lessen the amount of oestrogen needed to preserve bones – but this has yet to be confirmed.

Despite these new advances, prevention of osteoporosis is better than cure. Although it was previously claimed that exercise couldn't prevent osteoporosis once it had set in, new studies have shown that *regular exercise can help increase bone mass at any age.* In any case, we should all do as much as we can to strengthen our bones and reduce our risks of getting osteoporosis in the first place. See Chapter 6.

Heart Disease and HRT

Before the menopause, women's risk of heart disease is only one-fifth that of a man the same age. After it, the risk is the same. Heart disease is the leading cause of death in older women. If HRT could be shown definitely to protect against it, then that would indeed be a powerful reason to take it.

STUDYING THE STUDIES

For a start, most of the studies have been done in the United States and using a particular type of oestrogen (the 'conjugated' type derived from the urine of pregnant mares – see page 39). Another problem is the research itself. Some studies have been retrospective – i.e. looking back at patterns of heart disease among women who were on HRT – while others have been prospective – looking at groups of women over a period of time with the idea of finding out whether HRT is linked to heart disease. Some studies have examined women who have died of heart disease, others women with non-fatal types of the illness. Some have looked at healthy women, others women with existing evidence of heart disease. In consequence the results are highly contradictory and confusing.

Certainly oestrogen alone has been proved to confer protection against heart disease. The present consensus is that it can cut the coronary risk by up to 45 per cent. The biggest study so far, which looked at 48,470 American nurses over ten years, showed that taking oestrogen decreased the risk of coronary heart disease and deaths from heart disease. The treatment was not linked with any change in the risk of stroke. The researchers found that women who had never used oestrogen had twice the risk of suffering serious heart disease or a heart attack as did women who were taking oestrogen. So how might oestrogen help protect us against heart disease?

THE CHOLESTEROL CONNECTION

One fact that is known is that oestrogen affects blood fats. We all know by now the connection between coronary artery disease and high cholesterol levels in the blood. In fact the cholesterol story is not quite that straightforward either. Cholesterol is carried in the blood by substances called lipoproteins: high-density lipoprotein (HDL), sometimes known as 'good' cholesterol, carries cholesterol away from cells to the liver for disposal; low-density lipoprotein (LDL), sometimes known as 'bad' cholesterol, carries cholesterol to the cells. These LDLs can leave some cholesterol stuck to the artery walls, where it clogs them up, leading to narrowed arteries and the risk of a heart attack.

Oestrogen is thought to act as a protection by reducing levels of harmful LDLs in the bloodstream and raising levels of the beneficial HDLs. Before the menopause, women tend to have higher levels of 'good' HDL cholesterol in the blood, which is why it is thought they are at lower risk of heart attack.

But, of course, in women who haven't had a hysterectomy, any oestrogen taken has to be balanced by progestogen in order to avoid the risk of endometrial cancer. What isn't clear is whether adding progestogen counteracts the good done by the oestrogen. It's known that some types of progestogen increases the risk of damage to blood vessels and alters blood fat levels in favour of the harmful LDL-type of cholesterol. But the extent – both of the harmful effects and the women who will benefit most from the apparent protective benefits – is still a mystery. It seems to be a question of getting exactly the right balance of progestogen to oestrogen in order to maintain the beneficial effects of oestrogen while minimizing the potentially harmful effects of progestogen.

Nor does the story stop there. The two hormones also have an effect on another type of the blood fats – the triglycerides – which are a risk factor for heart disease, because they increase clotting. Triglyceride levels tend to be 'naturally' higher in people who are very overweight, or have an alcohol problem. They are also higher in diabetics and women on the Pill. Oestrogen boosts triglycerides, but progestogen actually lowers them. This means that giving the lowest possible dose of progestogen, in order to produce the most favourable pattern of LDLs and HDLs, has to be weighed against the risk of raising the levels of triglycerides. Again, more studies are needed urgently.

HIGH BLOOD-PRESSURE AND STROKES
The effects of HRT on raising or lowering the risk of high blood-

pressure and strokes are just as inconclusive. The combined contraceptive Pill (which contains oestrogen and progestogen) is known to cause high blood-pressure – but the doses used in HRT are much lower and of a different sort to those used in the Pill. On the other side of the coin, oestrogen widens the blood vessels – so is likely to lower blood-pressure. Yet oestradiol, a type of oestrogen used in HRT, can increase a protein produced by the liver called plasma renin substrate, which may increase blood-pressure. It's all very confusing.

Just to make matters even more complicated, the effects of the hormones may be determined by the way HRT is taken. The latest thinking is that giving HRT by implant or patch form, which avoids the first passage through the liver, may minimize the increase in plasma renin substrate. What is not known is whether this might then cancel out the other potential benefits.

At present, in some formulas of HRT different types of progestogen are being introduced which have weaker, opposing effects. However, it is not yet known whether these also have weaker effects on the lining of the uterus and so are weaker in fighting the risk of endometrial cancer. The $64,000 question is whether HRT in patch or implant form is as beneficial as the pill form in terms of preventing heart disease. If they are, some of the possible harmful side-effects may be avoided, but at the same time the beneficial effects may be cut too. As always it's far from simple.

Although the weight of evidence seems at present to be in favour of HRT, we need more good, controlled trials before we will have any definitive answers. Unfortunately there are no screening procedures that will measure your risk of contracting heart disease. So it's up to you to weigh up your own risks, then in consultation with your specialist decide whether HRT is right for you.

Am I at Risk?

The three main risk factors for heart disease are:

1. High blood cholesterol levels

   You are more likely to have raised blood cholesterol levels if you are overweight, and especially if you are an 'apple' i.e. carry weight around your belly rather than in your hips and thighs (a 'pear'). Other factors which can raise cholesterol levels include smoking, continual stress, and a diet high in saturated fats.

2. Continual high blood-pressure

   Constant high blood-pressure can damage the delicate lining of the arteries, causing a build up of cholesterol. Strokes in particular are linked with high blood-pressure.

3. Smoking

   Smoking causes the body to release hormones such as adrenalin, and makes the blood stickier and likelier to clot, and also temporarily raises blood-pressure. The carbon-monoxide in cigarettes reduces the amount of oxygen in the blood.

Other risk factors are:

● Family history

   If your father had a heart attack before the age of 50 or if your mother had one before 55.
● Diabetes
● Lack of exercise
● Stress
● Overweight

If you are on HRT you should have blood-pressure checks every six months. If your blood-pressure rises significantly, you should discuss with your doctor whether you should come off the treatment or change to another brand. If you develop severe headaches, or if you notice any unusual symptoms such as blurred vision, weakness, numbness in any part of your body or unusual pains in your chest, you should see the doctor. It's also a good idea to have your blood glucose and cholesterol levels checked from time to time. And of course, you must try to maintain a healthy lifestyle, with plenty of exercise and a diet low in fats and high in fibre (as outlined in Chapter 6).

CHAPTER FOUR

HRT *for Emotional Symptoms*

'When I went through my menopause I suffered terribly from hot flushes. But the worst thing of all was the complete change from being a happy person to being depressed. I used to burst into tears for no reason, I didn't want to do anything or go anywhere. From being someone who used to look forward to going to work and going out I became a recluse. I didn't know what had happened. I became argumentative at work: if the boss asked me to do something I would think, "Why should I?" And I began to forget things: people's names, things I was doing. I would be halfway upstairs and think "What am I coming up here for?"

'This lasted about a year and a half until I went on HRT. It transformed my life. The flushes cleared up, and I found so much energy, I was able to start swimming and running again. I started a swimming club at work and had my own water polo team. I took up weight training and running. Everyone commented on how much happier and energetic I was.'

HELEN, 54

'I started going through the most terrible menopause. I was dizzy and my memory was going to pot. I had to write everything down before I forgot it. I thought I was going senile. I really took it out on my family: my poor husband suffered terribly.

'As soon as I went on HRT everything cleared up fantastically. The physical symptoms were the first to get better. I started taking it on Thursday and by Monday I felt the difference. My memory took a long time to come back, but that feeling of well-being came back within a month.'

KILMENY, 45

One of the biggest controversies raging around HRT is whether it can help with the emotional symptoms of the menopause. For a start there is argument about whether such symptoms exist at all. One study reported in the *Lancet* (1987) found that 86 per cent of menopausal women suffered from clinical psychiatric illness, and a high proportion suffered from clinical depression. However, consultant psychiatrist Dr Barbara Ballinger gives short shrift to this idea, saying: 'The physical changes of the menopause have little impact on mental health. There is simply no evidence that psychological disorder increases after menstrual periods stop. There is,' she adds, 'some evidence . . . to suggest a very small increase in psychological disorder in the five years *before* menstruation stops, but the cause of this is ill-understood. The idea that the menopause itself causes psychological and emotional disturbances is a myth and must be abandoned.'

Fair enough, but what of those women who do feel they are living on an emotional roller coaster? Is it because of their hormones? Or is it to do with other factors in their lives? The truth is we don't really know, but the myths surrounding the menopause make it all too easy for emotional problems cropping up at this time to be attributed to the change of life.

The 'popular' picture of the menopausal woman is one who is tense, anxious and snappy, or forever bursting into tears. On the other hand, we've all read about those lucky (mythical?) creatures who 'sail through' the change of life with nary a change in step. Does that mean they didn't have any problems? Or did they just keep quiet about them? Were they the sort of people who rise above difficulties and always look on the bright side? Were they simply too busy to notice? What are we to make of it all?

One thing that is certain is that changes in mood and emotion are normal reactions to any kind of upheaval. Just which emotions can be linked to the internal changes taking place, and which ones are unrelated, is difficult to ascertain.

As with premenstrual syndrome, a bewildering number of emotional symptoms can be laid at the door of the menopause. According to one survey, carried out by nurse Joyce Masling, these symptoms include: nervous tension, irritability, mood swings, sleep problems, over-tiredness, lethargy and loss of energy, loss of confidence, an inability to concentrate, and depression – this last symptom caused by the thought of approaching old age, the end of the childbearing years, a reduction of family responsibilities, and, intriguingly, 'other reasons'. Lack of interest in sex, irritating memory lapses and absentmindedness are other commonly reported complaints. One woman told me how she put the milk in the airing cupboard! Another recalled how she would go to a meeting at work and forget what she wanted to say.

The danger of blaming such symptoms simply on the 'change of life' in the same way as the same symptoms earlier in life are often attributed to 'premenstrual syndrome' or 'postnatal depression' is that this can prevent us from examining aspects of our lives that we might like to change and that might in truth be responsible for these emotions.

The menopause, like giving birth, tends to be seen as an illness in our society. So when a woman goes to her doctor complaining of emotional disturbance, the doctor is faced with the dilemma, 'Is it a psychiatric illness (clinical depression) or a result of the menopause?' Val Godfree and Malcolm Whitehead outline the scenario in their book for doctors *HRT: Your Questions Answered*:

'The symptoms of "depressed mood" . . . when combined with other symptoms such as feelings of worthlessness, anxiety, crying, fatigue, loss of drive, aches and pains, headaches etc . . . is suggestive of clinical depression.'

However, they admit that, 'In most cases the problems presented by perimenopausal women are less severe and not continuous but fluctuating. Therefore, their depression is a symptom and rarely part of a true affective disorder.'

In other words, you aren't going mad! So why are you feeling emotionally unsettled – and can HRT help? As always there are several possible explanations.

It's Your Hormones

Enthusiasts of HRT often attribute the feelings of depression, lack of energy, irritability and so on to lack of oestrogen. First they surmise that the physical effects of the menopause, such as night sweats and so on, which *are* caused by waning oestrogen levels, can have a 'domino' effect: i.e., constantly waking up drenched in sweat leads to disturbed sleep, which in turn results in tiredness, fatigue, snappiness and the feeling that life just isn't worth living.

Another theory that is gaining in popularity is the idea that a shortage of oestrogen actually has a direct effect on the central nervous system. Researchers have discovered oestrogen receptors in the brain, which, according to Drs Godfree and Whitehead, 'appear to be concentrated in those areas currently believed to be associated with emotion.'

According to this view, HRT *can* help with emotional problems, either by removing the physical symptoms that are leading to the emotional ones, or by acting directly as a 'mental tonic'.

Feeling All Washed Up

Other writers on the menopause take the view that the emotional upheavals are more connected to the way menopause and older women are seen in our society. Nurse Joyce Masling sums up this viewpoint in an article in *Nursing Times* (September 1988):

> 'In our society, the menopause tends to be seen as a negative event. It is the end of the childbearing years, with children growing up and becoming independent and women with no children may regret that now there is no further chance of having a baby. A woman may regret all the opportunities she has missed or the things she has not achieved and feel that it is now too late.
>
> 'The emphasis today is on youth and physical attractiveness, and the ageing menopausal woman may look in the mirror and feel depressed and unattractive, forgetting that she has many other qualities of maturity and experience to offer which are not yet developed in a younger woman. Then, too, her husband may be preoccupied with his career and spend time away from home.'

Phyllis, 58, describes her experience:

> 'There were psychological reasons for feeling dreary, as I did. You have arrived at the point where you feel you're never going to have choices over your body anymore. You know you're never going to have more children. Round about 45 there's a great cliff and some people fall over it. I managed to cling on, but the next thing is you feel you start to look your age. A lot of my contemporaries went into a permanent greyness at this age, I noticed. Those that didn't became over-cheerful in a way that felt false to me.

'My husband was at the peak of his career, and the children were off to university. Suddenly I was almost entirely alone. I was worried and depressed while I worked it out. I thought about it and decided there were two things I could do: I had the chance for the first time to do things on my own, or I could sit back and become one of those women who lives for her husband and children and becomes rather dull. I didn't want to do that, so I looked at all the things I was moderately interested in and singled out one (I was lucky enough not to have to go out to work). In the end, the menopause transformed me. But when my sister went through it, she was not transformed.'

None of us is immune to negative images of the change of life. In a society that places as high a value on youth and beauty as ours does, it's all too easy to see loss of periods as the beginning of the end, rather than, potentially, the end of the beginning. And it's hardly surprising if these attitudes gradually chip away at our self-esteem and confidence – especially if we're feeling lousy physically. Indeed, some intriguing research reported by psychologist Dr Myra Hunter in *Your Menopause: Prepare Now for a Positive Future* shows that women who are depressed before the menopause actually report more hot flushes and other physical symptoms. So finding ways to beat depression before you hit the change of life could actually improve your health and well-being and reduce the need for HRT or treatment for depression later on.

Many of those who favour this theory about the causes of menopausal misery question the value of HRT in helping to combat it. After all, if the symptoms are caused by dis-satisfaction with life, or age-ist attitudes on the part of those around us, taking hormones isn't going to cure them, as 'agony aunt' Claire Rayner argues in her book, *Woman*:

'Women need to be sure that when they have problems in their forties and fifties they are correctly identifying the causes.

No One to Talk to

Negative images of the menopause plus feelings of isolation contribute to many of the symptoms of depression, as Amanda, 32, who underwent a premature menopause, points out.

'There was no one I could talk to, even my mother hasn't had her menopause yet. At first I denied it was happening. I didn't have my IUD taken out, but then my uterus shrank so much it actually expelled it. I couldn't bring myself to start HRT. When I read the blurb on the packet saying, "Now you've reached the change of life," I refused to believe it applied to me.

'It imposed an enormous strain on my marriage, because David had the same problems as me coming to terms with it. We had no sex life, and we couldn't discuss it. I think because I'm so young I questioned it more than someone going through it later. I was very aware of the prejudice against menopausal women and the way people make jokes about the menopause.

'A lot of marriages end when women reach their menopause and men make jokes about menopausal women. Others belittle it by saying, "It's only the menopause, for goodness sake, get on with it" But in fact it's the most difficult thing I've ever had to cope with because it relates to your whole identity.'

Amanda found that throwing herself into her work helped.

'I went through definite stages of grief – numbness, anger, depression. Finally I changed my job to one nursing children with cancer. I got promoted and one day I woke up and found the anguish gone.'

It isn't reasonable to blame your hormones when it's your home or your husband or your housework or your hatred of your job that is to blame. And it's surely foolish to think that taking a potentially risky drug like oestrogen is going to relieve such feelings.'

Am I at Risk?

Claire Rayner goes on to describe some South African research which pinpoints risk factors that it is particularly likely you will suffer disagreeable symptoms at the menopause. The first is 'psychosomatic responsiveness' – whether or not you tend to develop physical symptoms as a result of emotional stress. For example, when you are worried or under stress, do you often get headaches, nausea, diarrhoea, and so on?

The second risk factor is your level of 'personal life satisfaction'. Are you basically happy with your life, your job, your family, and the way your life has gone so far? If you aren't, then menopause, being a turning point, may trigger off feelings of discontent and unhappiness.

'I do think your mental attitude and approach has to do with how you cope with the menopause. One of the things I am sure that brought on my depression was leaving university, where I had been studying for four years as a mature student. All of a sudden I had nothing to do every day and it affected my mental attitude. Since I have been helping my husband with his medical practice, I have a new and more worthwhile role and I feel much better.'

LUCINDA, 55

The third factor is your view of the two sexes. If your view of what is womanly and what is manly are very set and stereotyped, you may find it difficult to adjust once a major part of your female role – i.e. childbearing – is no longer possible. This combined with the negative attitudes towards older women inherent in our society may again spark off depression.

Research has also shown that certain people are particularly vulnerable to reacting to life's knocks with depression. These include:

- those who have previously suffered mental or emotional problems,
- those who don't have someone in whom they feel they can confide, such as a partner, relative or close friend,
- those who find any sort of change difficult and anxiety-provoking.

This doesn't mean you are to blame if you get depressed, but it can be a pointer to the need to prepare yourself in advance for the challenges of the menopause, and if you are already going through it to establish support networks and other means of helping yourself cope.

Not in the Mood

What about lack of interest in sex – one of the most commonly quoted 'emotional difficulties' of the menopause? As we saw in Chapter 1, this can be related to the physical difficulties caused by a dry vagina, which makes lovemaking uncomfortable. On the other hand, lack of interest in sex is often quoted as a symptom of depression. Treat the depression and desire returns.

Some commentators, however, say that loss of sexual responsiveness may be related more to hiccups in a marriage or relationship than to physical or mental problems. Psychiatrist Dr Barbara Ballinger, quoted in an article in the *Independent* (October 1991) says:

'In other words, what the husband or partner perceives to be loss of libido [in his wife] may be [a] lack of interest in him, with the menopause being used by his wife as an excuse for avoiding sexual contact.'

She adds that assessing a woman's sex drive is difficult because frequency of intercourse is often still determined by the man.

In another study, carried out by psychologist Dr Myra Hunter, other factors were linked with a decline in sexual interest, such as being under stress, having marital problems, ill health, negative attitudes to the menopause, as well as severe hot flushes or vaginal dryness.

Vaginal dryness, as seen in Chapter 2, does respond to HRT, but it may be too much to expect other sexual problems to clear up miraculously once you start taking hormones. It could be that counselling is what you need.

Finally, the menopause might even improve your sex life. Myra Hunter's research showed that 84 per cent of post-menopausal women were satisfied with their sexual relationships, compared with 81 per cent of pre-menopausal ones.

The Happiness Pill?

The argument that oestrogen may help with mental symptoms is a complicated one, because of the known power of the 'placebo effect'. A certain proportion of people will get better no matter what treatment they are given. It's a testament to the power of the mind: we get better because we expect to do so. Another factor is that women attending a menopause clinic often find themselves being listened to and taken seriously for the first time. The enormous power of feeling that you are not alone should not be underestimated. Just knowing you have a sympathetic listener can do much to relieve mental stress – with or without the hormones.

However, there are convincing studies showing that irritability, fatigue, anxiety and depression can be counteracted by oestrogen. For example, in a study of 64 patients reported by Drs Godfree and Whitehead, oestrogen was found to be more effective than a placebo in alleviating hot flushes, insomnia and vaginal dryness, as well as irritability, poor memory, anxiety, worry about age and worry about oneself; it also increased optimism and good spirits. In an attempt to see whether the 'domino effect' mentioned above was coming into play, the researchers then re-examined the accounts of 20 patients who hadn't reported hot flushes, and found that poor memory, anxiety, and worry about age and self were still lessened by oestrogen. So it seems that oestrogen can lift mood on its own, irrespective of its effect on physical symptoms.

Another factor is that oestrogen improves sleep. Studies have shown that the drug lessens the amount of time it takes to drop off at night (what experts call the sleep latency period), and also increases REM (rapid eye movement) sleep, during which we dream. Anyone who has ever experienced prolonged periods of sleep deprivation, perhaps when looking after a young baby, will know how ratty you feel the next day, and how difficult it is to concentrate. It's even thought that some cases of postnatal depression are related to constantly interrupted, unsatisfying sleep. So, by making for sounder sleep, oestrogen may lead to a less agitated mind. (If you don't want to or can't take HRT, there are plenty of other things you can try to help you get a more peaceful night: see Chapter 6.)

Unfortunately, as we've seen time and again with HRT, it's not quite as straightforward as all this sounds, because even if oestrogen does help you feel more positive mentally, the progestogen factor may counteract these benefits. For while oestrogen may well act as a mental tonic, progestogen may have disagreeable psychological side-effects. The list of these, as quoted by Drs John Stevenson and Mike Marsh in an article in the doctors' newspaper *Pulse* (February 1992), include:

- aggression
- irritability
- anxiety
- restlessness
- panic attacks
- depressed mood
- moodiness
- poor concentration
- forgetfulness
- lethargy

Sound familiar? It's almost identical to the symptoms listed in Chapter 2 as characteristic of the menopause. Not all women experience these side-effects; however, women who have suffered badly from PMS (premenstrual syndrome) seem more likely to suffer, perhaps because they are 'vulnerable' in some way to progesterone. Changing to a lower dose of progestogen or to a different type of progestogen may sometimes solve the problem, but not always.

Addicted to Feeling Good?

Another worrying question is whether oestrogen is addictive. Doctors experienced in using HRT have observed a curious phenomenon. Some women who have had implants inserted return for another one before the time expected, even though the levels of oestrogen in their blood are within the normal range. As time goes on they need ever more frequent doses to enable them to feel better. By then they may be experiencing symptoms of oestrogen overdose – sore breasts, nausea and fluid retention. Eventually they are returning every few weeks as opposed to every six months for a top-up of the drug.

The problem (known medically as tachyphylaxis) is one that principally affects women who have been treated with the implant-type of HRT, however Drs Godfree and Whitehead observe, 'we suspect [it] may occur with other routes of administration.' For these unlucky women, the only solution is to submit to a period of 'cold turkey' which, as Godfree and Whitehead admit, can be 'long, slow and uncomfortable'.

Quite why HRT has this effect on some women and not on others is yet another of the unanswered questions about HRT. It is thought that those who have undergone premature menopause (and who are therefore more likely to have implants) or who have a history of previous mental problems are more likely to be at risk.

What are we to conclude from all this? Again, the questions raised are complex and as yet we really haven't any firm answers. What seems likely is that menopausal depression will turn out to result from a mixture of all the factors mentioned, as Dr Sadja Greenwood points out in her book *Menopause the Natural Way*:

'Our psychology – our moods, our outlook on life – is affected by the world around us *and* by our inner biology. The interactions between all these factors are so intimate that it is artificial to try to separate them. During the menopausal years the body goes through a major transition which is experienced differently by every woman, depending on her general health, her body awareness, and the rate at which her hormone levels drop. Her psychological reactions to this transitional phase will be determined by both her biochemistry and her outer circumstances. Each affects the other – inner and outer worlds are inseparable and in constant interaction.'

Having considered all the arguments, if you do decide to take HRT to help you get through emotional difficulties as you go through your menopause, you must do so in a realistic knowledge of what you can expect to achieve. HRT *may* help your memory and enable you to feel more relaxed and cheerful. But if at root your problems are to do with your feelings about the loss of youth, for example, HRT will do nothing to hold back the clock (despite the glamorous actresses who are used to promote it). If your depression is to do with your poor relationship with your partner, or a feeling that you haven't achieved anything in life, then HRT can't alter these, either. And even if you decide on taking HRT and find it helps, you need actively to work on improving your self-esteem and confidence so that you don't become unduly reliant on the 'high' produced by the hormones.

CHAPTER FIVE

Is It *for* Me?

'Our knowledge of HRT is much too patchy to allow
us to become wholesale purveyors of HRT to all
women over 45.'

FRANK LOEFFLER, Consultant Obstetrician and
Gynaecologist, St Mary's Hospital, London

'Should all women receive an offer of HRT? Yes –
probably.'

DR VAL GODFREE, Deputy Director of
the Amarant Centre, London

As the quotes above show, while some doctors believe every
woman should go on HRT at the menopause, others argue that,
as we are dealing with a potentially powerful drug with as
yet largely unknown long-term effects, only those suffering
troublesome symptoms should consider it. So is it right for you?
This chapter contains information to help you weigh up the
benefits against the risks. Because of this it may make somewhat
gloomy reading. However, it is important to have a realistic
knowledge of all the pros and the cons before you can be
expected to take an informed decision.

Questions Which Might Help You Decide

- Have you any specific personal risk factors, e.g. for osteoporosis, heart disease, breast cancer?
- How disruptive are your symptoms? (Keeping a diary may help you answer this one.)
- What can you do to reduce the effects of the menopause? (See Chapter 6.)
- What else can you do to look after your health?
- What are the risks of HRT?
- What other things are going on in your life right now that might be contributing to symptoms or making them worse?
- What sort of help are you getting from friends and family? Could they do more?
- Have you any friends who are going through the same experience, or are there any menopause groups nearby where you can go and talk?

'I Think I Might Give It a Try'

HRT is worth considering if:

- You have had a premature menopause naturally or as a result of medical treatment (see below).
- You have a strong family history of osteoporosis, or if you many of the risk factors associated with osteoporosis (page 60) apply to you, or if a bone scan has shown that you are at risk of osteoporosis.
- You are suffering badly with hot flushes and night sweats and they are interfering with your life to the extent that you feel unable to cope with them.
- You are experiencing severe vaginal dryness or frequent vaginal infections.

If you fall into any of these categories, first think about whether your symptoms are really due to the menopause. Keep a diary to try and identify what triggers symptoms and what, if anything, makes them better. If you dislike the idea of HRT, you might like to try other solutions such as the self-help and alternative therapies suggested in Chapter 6. However, if your symptoms are making your life miserable and there are no medical reasons why you *shouldn't* take HRT (see below), it might be worth a try.

If you are taking HRT to prevent osteoporosis, bear in mind that it needs to be taken for at least five years and preferably ten to be beneficial. And no matter what your reason for deciding to take HRT, it's particularly important to get the right treatment for you. If you aren't happy with the type of HRT prescribed after giving it a fair try (usually about three months), go back and ask if a change of method or dosage might help. *Persevere until you find the right combination for you, and remember that if you aren't happy with your doctor you can ask for a second opinion.* You'll find a list of menopause clinics in the Useful Addresses section of this book.

PREMATURE MENOPAUSE

One group of women who can definitely be helped by HRT are those who have undergone premature menopause, or premature ovarian failure (POF), to use the medical term. Such women are seven times more at risk of heart disease, and are also at extra risk of osteoporosis: a woman who undergoes the menopause at 30 will have the bones of a 70 year old by the time she is 50. In the mental Filofax we carry round in our heads, most of us pencil in the word menopause at around age 50, yet one in 20 women experiences the change of life before she hits her forties.

Psychologist and author Dr Myra Hunter, who carried out a study of reactions of prematurely menopausal women, says, 'Reactions depend on a woman's age and life experience, but all have to go through a period of grief and mourning. Younger women feel it is a burden they have to carry. They worry about telling boyfriends. Even those who never wanted children find the loss of their fertility painful. Those who already have children tend to be more worried about the physical effects and its impact on their looks. Anxieties about femininity and loss of self-confidence are common.'

Unfortunately, POF frequently goes unnoticed by doctors simply because they are not looking for it. A survey carried out by Dr Tim Spector of 5,000 women in four London doctors' practices found that less than a quarter of women who had gone through the menopause (whether early or nearer the average age) had received any HRT treatment – and those who had experienced premature menopause could certainly be considered much more in need of HRT to prevent problems such as osteoporosis and heart disease. (It's thought that the small increased risk of breast cancer HRT-users face doesn't apply to younger women because the hormones are merely putting them back to normal, so the risk is no greater than usual.)

WHAT CAUSES POF?
Just why some women's ovaries give out so much earlier than usual is still a mystery, although several explanations have been advanced.

Too Few Eggs
Each of us is endowed with around two to three million eggs at birth, but natural wastage means that by the time of the first period there are some three-to-four hundred thousand left. In fact, 99.9 per cent of eggs never mature sufficiently to be ovulated.

For reasons that aren't fully understood, but which may be genetic, some women are born without the full quota, so their eggs run out early.

Chromosomal Causes
Faulty chromosomes, and in particular a disease called Turner's

syndrome in which the second female X chromosome is missing, can lead to primary POF (when you never ovulate at all) or secondary POF (when you ovulate but stop early).

The Auto-immune Connection

There is also a theory that some auto-immune mechanism is at work by which the body attacks and destroys its own ovaries. A clue lies in the fact that other auto-immune illnesses such as thyroid disease, rheumatoid arthritis and adrenal failure are often linked to premature menopause.

We all possess antibodies that protect us against disease by coming into action when the body is attacked by an invader. For some reason, the body sometimes 'overreacts' and attacks its own tissues. It's now known that the body is capable of attacking its own ovarian tissue, blocking the production of eggs. The ovaries become encased in scar tissue, which prevents them from developing and prevents ovulation from occurring. One expert says, 'Seven out of ten POF sufferers show auto-antibodies which suggests some such process is taking place. It is a leap but I suspect auto-immunity will be found to lie at the root of the majority of POF.'

Medical Treatment

Pelvic surgery for other gynaecological conditions can be responsible for POF. Hysterectomy, even without the removal of the ovaries, leads to premature menopause in over a third of cases.

The uterus is supplied with nourishment and oxygen by two blood vessels – the ovarian artery and the uterine artery. The uterine artery is cut back with the removal of the womb, and this disrupts the blood supply to the ovaries, causing them to wither and die. Pelvic surgery for other gynaecological conditions such as endometriosis or cysts sometimes cuts off the blood supply to the ovaries. And chemotherapy and radiation therapy for certain types of cancer, such as leukaemia, is another cause.

The Lifestyle Factor

Many American doctors believe environmental and lifestyle factors play a part in POF. Infections such as mumps are to blame in some cases. Smokers tend to go into menopause earlier because chemicals in cigarettes stunt egg development. Heavy drinking is known to affect the ovaries, too. Although many cases of POF are discovered when a woman comes off the Pill, it isn't thought that the Pill is the cause, simply that it masks the condition.

As for other environmental factors, the experts admit they are still in the dark. Doctors Michael Alper, Peter Garner and Machelle Seibel, however, who have researched POF in the United States, suggest: 'It is possible that chemicals in our diet and environment will prove toxic to follicular development, and that in susceptible individuals various drugs, toxins and viruses cause POF.'

COPING WITH POF

Menopausal symptoms are often more severe with POF, and especially in those women whose menopause has been surgically induced. However, not all sufferers experience symptoms. Lucy, 40, who underwent premature menopause six years ago, said, 'I never experienced hot flushes or anything. I've always felt completely healthy.'

Others are less fortunate. A family therapist who runs menopause groups says, 'Coming to terms with it involves learning to let go of what might have been and beginning to value what you are. All the special things about you are still the same, but that is hard to believe when you are newly bereaved, as these women are. It also means reclaiming your sexual identity and separating it from the reproductive function.'

Talking to other women who have had similar experiences helps. Another women decided to take a part-time catering course with a view to opening a restaurant; 'In the back of my mind I'd always put off doing anything like that "just in case" I had a baby. Having the menopause was hard, but it forced me to concentrate on what I wanted to do with the rest of my life.'

There are ways of overcoming childlessness, of course, though these can be difficult and expensive, and you may not end up with a child in the end. Adoption is one possibility, but be prepared to persevere, as babies are scarce. And the technique of ovum donation, using IVF – *in vitro* fertilization, the 'test-tube baby' technique – enables some women to become mothers. HRT can help make the lining of the uterus more receptive to the implantation of an egg. However, IVF treatment is only available in one or two NHS hospitals, and private infertility treatment is not cheap.

Premature menopause can symbolize a loss of control over life. Anything that enables you to take control and to value what you have can help. For example, exercise and vitamins put you back in the driver's seat. Some women throw themselves into work, focussing on the positive advantages of having more time to devote to their career than women who are juggling work and family. Others learn to value the extra freedom to have holidays and visit places they could never have gone with children.

'I'm not Sure If It's for Me'

At one time doctors were rightly extremely cautious about prescribing HRT, and there were a whole host of medical conditions which were thought to rule it out. Today's preparations of 'natural' oestrogens have changed all that, and many doctors now feel much happier about prescribing HRT where previously it would have been contraindicated. Below I list the definite contraindications and the ones where you need to give the matter careful thought and decide in consultation with a specialist experienced in HRT.

DEFINITELY NOT
There are certain definite medical reasons why some women shouldn't take HRT.

Undiagnosed Vaginal Bleeding

There are many causes for this, but because it could be a sign of cancer of the uterus or cervix it's important to get it checked out before going on HRT.

You should have an internal vaginal exam, cervical smear and D & C to check the lining of the uterus.

Pregnancy

It's easy to confuse pregnancy with the irregular bleeding that often heralds the menopause. And while it's thought that the levels of oestrogen and progestogen contained in HRT are so low that there could be no adverse effect on a foetus, there are fears that certain types of progestogen could stimulate the development of male characteristics if the unborn baby were exposed to them at a critical time in its development.

Breast Cancer or a Strong Family History of Breast Cancer

This is yet another controversial area. Some types of breast cancer are oestrogen-dependent, and there is a risk that HRT may trigger off a recurrence. However, some consultants in some specialist breast cancer units say the risks are not proved, and are experimenting with giving HRT to women with breast cancer who are also experiencing severe menopausal symptoms. If you do decide to take the risk, you should do so in a full knowledge of the pros and cons (for a fuller discussion see page 98).

For the same reason it's also worth thinking very carefully before you take HRT if there is a strong family history of breast cancer (i.e. your mother or sister developed it before the age of 50).

Endometrial Cancer

Cancer of the lining of the womb is another oestrogen-dependent cancer. It's not known whether there's an increased risk of recurrence if you take HRT, because the necessary studies haven't been carried out. However, experts believe it's best to avoid HRT just in case.

If any of these conditions apply to you, the advice on alternatives in Chapter 6 may be particularly helpful.

THINK TWICE

The next group of conditions are slightly more woolly. Doctors often used to see them as contraindications, and some still do. However, in the light of current research, some of them might even be *indications* for taking HRT. You therefore need to think especially carefully about the pros and cons.

Previous Endometrial Hyperplasia

Endometrial hyperplasia is an overgrowth of the tissues of the lining of the womb. This condition, which if untreated can lead on to cancer, happens as a result of oestrogen stimulation, so HRT is not recommended. However, the situation is slightly more complicated because some reports have actually suggested that HRT may reverse some types of this condition. A hysterectomy is likely to be recommended, after which there is no further risk and it is safe (and, many doctors would argue, desirable) to take HRT.

Cervical and ovarian cancers haven't been shown to be linked to HRT. However, there have been some worrying reports that women who develop the rare type of ovarian cancer called endometroid ovarian cancer have a higher risk of developing tumours if they are taking HRT.

Heart Disease, High Blood-pressure or Blood-clots

Existing or previous heart disease, high blood-pressure or blood-clotting (thromboembolic) disease of the arteries or veins, or a family history of heart disease, must all be taken into consideration before beginning any treatment.

It used to be thought that HRT increased the risks of heart disease. However, as we saw in Chapter 3 this is no longer the case, and therapy may actually help protect against heart disease. You need to attend a specialist menopause clinic where you can weigh up the pros and cons, and must come to a decision in conjunction with your heart specialist.

Oestrogen can sometimes spark off high blood-pressure, though this is rare. If you suffer from the condition and it is under control, then it's safe to start therapy, though of course the doctor will want to keep a careful eye on you and adjust the dose if it appears to be having an effect on your blood-pressure. Some doctors believe the implant method may be better for high blood-pressure sufferers, though this hasn't been proved.

Thrombosis is slightly more complicated because of the risk that oestrogens may increase clotting. Your doctor may suggest using implants rather than patches or pills, as implants appear to minimize the risk. However, if you have developed thrombosis early in pregnancy or while you were taking the Pill, you could be oestrogen-sensitive, in which case you would need to visit a specialist menopause clinic where tests to determine your clotting factor can be performed.

Otosclerosis

Otosclerosis is a disease of the middle ear that causes progressive deafness.

There have been reports of the condition going downhill rapidly in those on oestrogen. On the other hand, some women don't experience any deterioration despite being on HRT for a long time.

Diabetes

If you have suffered diabetes from childhood you have a higher risk of developing heart disease or disease affecting the blood vessels – which as we've seen may be helped by HRT. However, oestrogens and progestogens affect the way the body processes carbohydrates, so the doctor will want to keep a careful eye on you during the first few months of treatment.

SLE

SLE is systemic lupus erythematosus, a chronic disease that causes inflammation of connective tissue. It is also an auto-immune disease in which, for reasons that are not understood, the body turns against itself. The disease appears to be linked in some way to the female sex hormones, affecting nine times as many women of childbearing age as men. Because of this link and because SLE can cause other problems in the body, HRT is not advised as it may aggravate the condition. However, each case needs to be considered individually.

Active Liver Disease

Because it has to pass through the liver HRT may impose a dangerous extra burden on an organ already damaged by a disease such as severe hepatitis where liver function tests are abnormal. HRT in pill form is out for this reason. However, if you are suffering badly from menopause symptoms, your doctor may suggest trying an HRT patch.

Fibroids

Fibroids are non-cancerous growths in the uterine wall. Their precise cause is unknown but is thought to be linked to an abnormal reaction to oestrogen (they usually shrink after the menopause, when the oestrogen supply dwindles). However, if you go on HRT this shrinkage does not occur, and sometimes the fibroids may even grow bigger. If you decide to take the risk and this happens, you will either have to give up the HRT or have a hysterectomy and take oestrogen alone. The decision is yours.

Gallstones

Taking HRT in pill form changes the composition of bile in a way that may increase the risk of gallstones forming. Some studies show that other forms of HRT such as patches and implants may be carry less risk, but again you need to weigh up the risks and benefits in consultation with the doctor before opting for HRT.

Endometriosis

If you have ever suffered this debilitating and painful condition, in which fragments of the womb lining grow in other parts of the pelvis, causing severe pain, think very carefully before taking HRT. Because the condition is oestrogen-dependent, going on HRT may start it up again. Even if you have had surgery there may still be tiny fragments of tissue left behind which can grow under the influence of the extra oestrogen.

A further group of conditions may be aggravated by HRT. If you suffer with any of these, again you should discuss it with your medical advisor:

- Epilepsy
- Migraine

    This can be broken down into *menstrual* migraine, which starts a day or two before your period and which may be a result of the fall in oestrogen levels at this time, and *premenstrual* migraine, which comes on four or five days before your period and which may be related to higher progesterone levels, in which case HRT may worsen it, especially during the progestogen part of the treatment.

- Varicose veins

    HRT can sometimes bring on or worsen aching in veins. However it doesn't appear to affect bloodflow to the lower legs or to spark off thrombosis.

THE BREAST CANCER CONTROVERSY

Although HRT has been around for almost 40 years, there are still question marks about its safety. The principal concern is whether it increases the risk of breast cancer. Although this next section makes somewhat scary reading, it's important to face the facts before making your own decision. One doctor writing in the medical magazine *Pulse* goes so far as to say, 'That there is evidence to show that this may be the case [that HRT increases the risk of breast cancer] should render usage absolutely unacceptable, unless the patient agrees to take part in what amounts to a personal clinical trial of the possible carcino-genicity [cancer-causing potential] of HRT.'

The issue is complicated because breast cancer is the most common cancer in women, affecting one in twelve of us over the course of a lifetime, and the risks rise as we get older. What we do know is that breast cancer seems to be related in some way to exposure to high levels of oestrogen over a period of time. For example, women who began their periods early, who are overweight (and who therefore have higher levels of certain types of oestrogen), women who have their first baby late, and women who have a late menopause all run a higher risk. And although the risk of breast cancer increases with age, the *rate* of increase falls after the menopause, which suggests a lowering of risk with the waning supply of oestrogen. There are other risk factors too. Women with a strong family history (i.e. one or more close female relatives who developed the disease before the age of 50) carry a risk of between one in two and one in four of developing the disease. We still don't know how much each of these factors weigh in the final analysis.

The whole issue is such a minefield because as well as the factors in the table overleaf, the studies which have been done are contradictory. Some report a slight increase in the risk of breast cancer, others don't. What set the alarm bells ringing were two studies carried out (in 1987 and 1989) which showed that HRT boosts the risk when taken from between five and nine years and six to ten years. *In other words, HRT doubles the risk of breast cancer when taken for ten years or more.*

Other cancer experts have refuted the evidence. Dr Trevor Powles, Consultant Physician at Britain's leading cancer hospital, The Royal Marsden, says: 'Half a million women have had the treatment [HRT] so far. If it did increase the risks there would have been a much bigger effect by now.' Some doctors believe that the progestogen part of HRT may actually protect the breast. This is based on the fact that progestogen discourages the division of cells in the lining of the womb, however whether or not this applies to breast tissue is uncertain, and some

Am I at Risk?

Many factors are involved in the development of breast cancer. You need to weigh up the various factors and see whether you think the possible added risk is worth it in your particular case.

Reliable studies show you are at higher risk of breast cancer if:

- a close relative contracted the disease before the age of 50, or if several female relatives – e.g. grand-mother, mother, aunt – had the disease
- you had an early start to your periods (12 or under) and have a late menopause (50 plus)
- you are overweight

Some studies show that your risk is increased if:

- you eat a high-fat diet
- you drink more than 14 units of alcohol a week (one unit is equivalent to one glass of wine, half a pint of beer or lager, a small glass of sherry or a measure of spirits)
- you have a history of benign breast disease
- you had your first child after the age of 30
- you were on the old-fashioned type of combined Pill for eight or more years when you were young

Some studies show your risk may be lowered if:

- you are vegetarian
- you don't drink alcohol
- you had your first child when you were young
- you breastfed for four years or more in total

evidence shows that progestogens actual increase cell division on breast tissue. In fact there is some evidence that the addition of progestogen may actually *boost* breast cancer risk. One breast cancer pioneer I interviewed for *She* magazine told me, 'If a woman said to me "I don't care what I die of, so long as it isn't breast cancer," I wouldn't prescribe her HRT.'

So the verdict is still in the balance. We still don't know whether it is the particular type of oestrogen prescribed that increases the risk (most of the studies have been done on the common 'conjugate equine oestrogens' derived from mare's urine). We don't know whether the increased risk rises with the length of time on HRT. And we don't know whether some women are more vulnerable to the dangers than others. Some studies suggest that women with a family history of breast cancer carry the highest extra risk, because they already have a predisposition to the disease. The genes load the gun; HRT may pull the trigger. Some studies have shown that oestrogen bumps up the breast cancer risk in women with 'benign' breast disease – but other studies have not found this to be the case.

We may soon have some answers to some of these questions. A major study of 30,000 breast cancer patients is currently being carried out by the Imperial Cancer Research Fund in Oxford, and is designed to settle the question once and for all when the results are published in 1994. The study will examine inter-national results of 40 previous studies and will clarify some of the issues. But the study is retrospective (i.e. looking back at previous studies), and before we can have any definite answers we still need good, well-designed trials using modern forms of HRT which take all the other risk factors mentioned into account.

The Cost-benefit Analysis

So where does all this leave you? The current medical thinking is that taking HRT for five years will protect against osteoporosis and heart disease without increasing the risk of breast cancer significantly. However, if you have any of the risk factors for breast cancer, as the evidence stands at present you may not be prepared to take any extra risks. You may prefer to avoid HRT and try other forms of treatment, orthodox or alternative, for the symptoms of the menopause. If you do decide not to take HRT, it's particularly vital to pay attention to measures you can take to preserve a healthy heart and bones.

On the other hand, you may believe that the risk of contracting breast cancer is one you would be prepared to take in order to take advantage of the potential benefits of HRT. Either way, the decision must be yours.

CHAPTER SIX

What Else Can I Do?

Self-help for Keeping Healthy

Staying healthy is vital if you intend to enjoy the rest of your life to the full – whether or not you decide to go on HRT. If you are fit both physically and mentally you will be in better shape to meet the challenges the menopause brings, whatever form they take.

The rules of good health are remarkably constant throughout life: eat a healthy diet, go easy on the alcohol, get enough exercise, develop close relationships and cultivate a positive outlook. But it's now more important than ever to stick to these rules. Interestingly, these same rules crop up time and again as ways of combating degenerative diseases and preventing premature ageing.

You Are What You Eat (and Drink)

A healthy diet is the cornerstone of good health at any age. Today (and for the first time this century) there's remarkable agreement about what constitutes the best diet for good health. Throughout the world the healthiest people follow three simple rules:

1. About half their food is made up of unrefined carbohydrates – starchy fibrous foods such as wholegrain breads, pasta, rice, potatoes, cereals.

Calcium-rich Foods

Cheddar cheese: 800 mg of calcium per 100 g
Semi-skimmed milk: 729 mg per 600 ml
Canned sardines: 550 mg per 100 g
Dried figs: 280 mg per 100 g
Milk chocolate: 220 mg per 100 g
Yoghurt: 195 mg per 100 g
Muesli: 190 mg per 100 g
Broccoli: 100 mg per 100 g
Prawns: 55 mg per 100 g
White wine: 14 mg per glass

2. They eat at least five portions of fruit and vegetables a day.
3. Their diet contains a minimum of saturated fat (found in animal products) – less than 10 per cent of their daily calorie intake – and some polyunsaturated and monounsaturated fat (found in vegetable oils) – between 3 and 7 per cent per day.

Once you hit the menopause your diet should also provide at least 1.5 grams of calcium a day – important for building strong bone (see box above) and for its natural calming and relaxing effect.

The kind of diet most experts recommend is lower in protein than the traditional 'meat and two veg' we have all been brought up on, but this is actually a good thing. A high-protein diet is linked with increased excretion of calcium in the urine, and may be a factor in the later development of osteoporosis. Your diet should also be low in sugar, as sugar has also been linked to greater losses of calcium, and naturally high in a range of vitamins that have been shown to combat specific menopausal problems, such as:

- Vitamin C (found in fruit and vegetables) is anti-infective and anti-stress.
- B-complex vitamins (found in cereals and egg yolk) are vital for a healthy nervous system and may help preserve a healthy vagina. Vitamins B_2 and B_6 have been shown to have oestrogen-like effects, and vitamin B_1 and pantothenic acid (another B vitamin) enhance the action of a type of oestrogen called oestradiol, though they have no oestrogenic activity themselves.
- Vitamin E (found in wheatgerm, soya beans, maize, and green, leafy vegetables) is beneficial in helping sweats and flushes, and dry vagina. It's thought to work by reducing the breakdown of progesterone.
- Beta carotene (found in red and yellow fruits and vegetables) helps fight cancer and heart disease. Vitamin A is also necessary for normal growth and strength of skin tissue, such as that of the vagina.
- Boron (a trace mineral found in apples, pears, tomatoes, prunes, raisins, dates, honey and milk) has been shown in trials to activate oestrogen and vitamin D (necessary for the absorption of calcium).

More controversial are vitamin supplements. Some experts argue that, so long as you are getting a good, balanced diet, there is no need for supplements. Others say that aspects of modern life such as pollution, pesticides, long storage times and processing methods deprive food of its natural goodness. What's more, allergies and food intolerance, plus encroaching age, mean we absorb vitamins and minerals from food less easily.

Be warned, however: high doses of vitamins can act as drugs, so it's best not to dose yourself. If you do decide to supplement your diet, beware of taking isolated vitamins and minerals, unless prescribed by a reliable practitioner, because of the danger of creating possible imbalances. Either take a good multi-vitamin and mineral complex such as *Gynovite* (which has been specially devised by an American gynaecologist for menopausal problems) or, best of all, consult an experienced nutritional practitioner who can tailor your treatment to your individual needs.

CAFFEINE

Too much caffeine not only keeps you awake at night, it can trigger flushes and has been found to induce a negative calcium balance, thus increasing the risk of osteoporosis. All good reasons to cut out − or at least to cut down on − tea, coffee, cola and other drinks containing caffeine. Soft drinks also tend to be loaded with chemicals called phosphates, which are linked with a higher loss of calcium from the urine. One menopause expert suggests restricting coffee and tea to before lunchtime and going for herbal teas, mineral water, juices and non-caffeinated drinks for the rest of the day.

ALCOHOL

The question of whether or not the odd tipple is harmful or helpful is a difficult one to answer. Most studies on the effects of alcohol have been done on men. Alcohol has different effects on women because of our different bodily make-up. However, recently several studies have been carried out which suggest powerful reasons to cut down on alcohol consumption if you can.

For a start, alcohol tends to leach oestrogen from the ovaries, and for this reason you may suffer more from symptoms such as flushes. Alcohol dilates the surface blood vessels, so may trigger a hot flush. Secondly, a heavy alcohol intake is a risk factor for osteoporosis, and in women with brittle bones, drinking too much can make you more liable to falls. Thirdly, some studies have shown that women who have a high alcohol intake are more at risk of breast cancer. All good reasons to stay off the bottle.

On the other hand, a study of British women reported in the *British Medical Journal* (January 1992) showed that *moderate* alcohol consumption (that is, less than two units a day) is linked with lower levels of the 'bad' LDL cholesterol and higher levels of the beneficial HDL cholesterol. What we don't know is whether this is directly due to the effects of alcohol or whether moderate drinkers have a healthier lifestyle generally and so are at lower risk of heart disease.

In the light of all this you may decide to give up drinking altogether, if you don't you should certainly aim to limit consumption to 14 units a week *maximum*.

Exercise

Exercise is vital to preserve the health of your heart and bones and to keep you supple. To do the bones any good the exercise you do must be 'gravity dependent'. Swimming is fine for developing suppleness and strength, but it isn't really that good for the bones, because the water holds your weight. Running, jogging, walking, dancing, skipping, tennis and so on all jar the bones slightly; this stimulates bone growth and calcification, so helping bones to become stronger.

In addition you need aerobic exercise, to strengthen the heart muscles. Until recently doctors recommended that we should all take vigorous exercise three times a week. This rule still holds good if you are motivated to keep at it. However, not many people stick with exercise programmes they find too demanding or intrusive, and it has recently been found that less strenuous exercise, such as walking, is just as beneficial *provided it is regular*. You won't feel the benefits as quickly with a slower paced exercise programme, but it is just as good for your bones and your heart.

Yoga is a particularly beneficial system of exercise. In a study carried out by the Yoga Biomedical Foundation, 83 per cent of women taking up yoga found it helped with menopausal problems.

Relationships

Throughout life our relationships change and develop as we pass through different stages. If you are in a long-term partnership and have children, it can be exciting to be able to spend time with your partner and learn to relate to each other again as individuals and not simply as parents. Scales of marital satisfaction rate the time when childbearing responsibilities are over as some of the most rewarding, and satisfaction scores which plummet on the birth of the first child rise again at this time.

Sometimes, of course, a relationship can fall casualty to these changes. Divorce rates show a slight upturn at this time – often because couples have been hanging on in an unsatisfactory relationship 'for the sake of the children'. Painful though any type of relationship break-up is, do remember there *is* life after divorce: many women who have been through the agony of splitting up say afterwards that it was also a time of growth and learning.

If you are on your own the menopause can be a time to evaluate the relationships you have, to discard those that aren't rewarding and nurture those in which there is a true feeling of intimacy and sharing. The presence of a close, confiding relationship is a proven depression-beater, but such a relationship doesn't have to be with a husband or partner, it can just as easily be with a friend or relative. Some women find joining a menopause group, where they can share their thoughts and experiences with other women who are at the same stage in life, helpful too.

Think Positive

In a world where youth is equated with sexual attractiveness and success, the realization that time is marching on can be a hard one. Older women may be at best invisible, at worst the butt of jokes and derogatory comments. Even high-profile older women are not exempt – unless of course they have managed to stay young-looking and glamorous. Difficult though it is, it's important not to take on board these negative images and to value ourselves for the maturity and experience we acquire with age. As the authors of *Menopause: A Time for Positive Change* comment:

'Many women say that after the age of 40 or so they suddenly feel as though they "dare" to do or say much more than before: they don't care so much what other people might think, and find that maturity brings them a confidence they never used to have as younger women.' Such a change of attitude might be a positive side to the 'invisibility' of older women.

It can't be emphasized too strongly that the menopause can be a time of positive change. If you have never had a career it can be a time to reassess the opportunities open to you, to find out about education and training. If you are already in work it might be time to think about a change of direction – about self-employment, for example. Alternatively, if you don't need to work for the money and you don't want a job, now is the time to take up new interests or develop old ones.

Alternatives to HRT?

Strictly speaking there are no alternatives to HRT, since none of the alternative therapies actually replace oestrogen. However, many alternative therapies are successful in treating the troublesome symptoms of the menopause, though their value in preventing long-term consequences such as osteoporosis and heart disease is more debatable. They can also be used to complement conventional therapy, so even if you decide to opt for HRT you may be able to get by with a lower dose if you combine it with one or more of the natural therapies.

HERBAL HELP

Herbs have been used for centuries to prevent and cure illness, and many herbs form the basis of modern drugs. Herbal treatment can be a useful alternative or complement to HRT or other conventional forms of therapy. In particular, certain plants known as phytoestrogens (plant oestrogens) are said to have an oestrogenic effect on the body, though not as powerful as that of HRT. They are said to have a balancing effect, restoring dwindling oestrogen levels in those with a shortage and lowering excess levels to normal in those with too much. This is why the same plant may be recommended by a herbalist for conditions due to too much oestrogen as for conditions due to too little. In their book *Encyclopedia of Natural Medicine*, American naturopaths Michael Murray and Joseph Pizzorno explain, 'If oestrogen levels are low, since phytoestrogens have some oestrogenic activity they will cause an increase in oestrogen effect; if oestrogen levels are high, since phytoestrogens bind to oestrogen-receptor binding sites, thereby competing with oestrogen, there will be a decrease in oestrogen effects.'

According to Murray and Pizzorno, herbs with a long history of oestogenic activity include dong quai (*Angelica sinensis*), liquorice (*Glycyrrhiza glabra*), unicorn root (*Aletris farinos*), black coholsh (*Cimicifuga racemosa*), Fennel (*Foeniculum vulgare*), and false unicorn root (*Helonias opulus*).

Another herb, chasteberry (*Agnus vitex castus*) has a reputation for its balancing effect on the reproductive system. In this case the effects are more like those of progestogen. A combination of, say, false unicorn root with chasteberry provides a kind of herbal HRT.

Herbal medicine alone cannot prevent osteoporosis, though a herbalist would look at your diet and exercise regimes.

As far as heart disease is concerned, there are several herbs that improve circulation. They include hawthorn, garlic, lime, motherwort, lily of the valley and horse chestnut.

Because these are all herbs with potentially powerful effects, you should always consult a qualified herbal practitioner rather than trying to go it alone.

'I originally went on HRT at the age of 52 because of "pains in my insides", hot flushes and feeling rather depressed and uncertain. HRT didn't cure the pains, but it did make me feel very lively. I didn't realize it was the HRT doing this until I came off it, I'd simply been grateful I was one of those people who had lots of "natural" energy.

'I was on HRT for three to four years when I was suddenly seized with pulmonary embolism and thrown into hospital. They could find no reason for it, and asked if I were taking anything. I said "Yes, HRT." The doctor ordered me to come off it immediately.

'When I came off HRT I felt really ghastly. I felt very tired and my energy level was lower. A doctor I know who practises herbal medicine (I'll call him "Dr A") said I should come and see him if I wanted to. I didn't want to go at first. One of the dilemmas of getting orthodox medical treatment is that you feel great you should stick with it even if it doesn't seem to be helping. But finally I went to see him. He explained for about half an hour what herbal medicines could do; he knew I was anxious about coming off *Warfarin* (a blood-thinning drug used to treat embolism). He gave me a bottle of the most revolting medicine – and I've been going to him ever since! One of the after-effects of embolism is a lot of leg pain. Dr A gave me some horse chestnut, which is a natural way of helping circulation, and my leg got better. I feel quite different as well, more confident. I don't know if it's the herbs or just having someone like Dr A to go and talk to, but in any case, I'm much less anxious and nervous.'

SUSIE, 58

HOMOEOPATHY
Homoeopathy works on the principle that 'like cures like'. Remedies made from plants, herbs, minerals and tissues are

used in microscopic dilutions to treat illness. The idea is that giving minuscule doses of a medicine that in a healthy person would produce symptoms of the condition being treated somehow stimulates the body's own healing mechanism.

Several scientific trials have proved the value of homoeopathy in treating conditions such as hay fever and fibromyalgia. There are no research studies on the effects of homoeopathic remedies on menopausal symptoms. There are, however, many anecdotal reports to suggest they can help. The homoeopath tries to match the symptom picture of the homoeopathic remedy to your individual symptoms.

Remedies can be used at two levels: as a first aid treatment for minor symptoms, and for various acute and chronic illnesses after the practitioner has talked to you in detail and found the right remedy for you. This is called constitutional prescribing.

It's common to experience an aggravation of symptoms when you first start taking a remedy (see below) – but this is usually a good sign, a proof that the remedy chosen is the right one.

Some homoeopathic remedies said to be especially useful for menopausal symptoms include:

- Sepia: For hot flushes with intense congestion of the face and throbbing in the head which is aggravated by heat.
- Natrum Mur: For complaints following a loss. Symptoms include nervous irritability, bursting headaches, dry mucous membranes, slow digestion, constipation.
- Lachesis: For headaches, flushes, tightness in the chest and fatigue. Complaints are worse on waking, worse on becoming warm; patient cannot breathe in the heat; patient often wakes from sleep with sense of suffocation and must sit up bent forward or rush to open the window.

If none of these suit you it's best to consult a homoeopath, who will prescribe a constitutional remedy. Homoeopaths are either lay people who have undergone an in-depth training or doctors who are also homoeopaths. Because of the long-term risks of osteoporosis you may prefer to consult a homoeopath who is also a doctor. The whole subject is extremely complex, as a qualified doctor and homoeopath I interviewed admits:

'HRT is marvellous for a few women, no good whatsoever for a few, and a few feel better on it. From a homoeopathic point of view you can get good results with short-term symptoms, but no research has been done on problems such as osteoporosis and heart disease. Osteoporosis is of course very serious, but a lot of women have HRT when they are not at risk just to be on the safe side, without having tests done which would show whether or not they are actually at risk of the disease.'

He adds: 'A lot of women feel unhappy about taking HRT, and from a totally unscientific view I must say I side with them. I can't help feeling that if the hormones stop they do so for a reason. The menopause isn't a deficiency disease in the same way as diabetes, in that diabetes is an illness: the diabetic can't live without insulin, whereas no one dies through lack of hormones. The most important feature is that it is self-limiting, and if you mask the symptoms with hormones you don't know when it has stopped. It is, however, very complex, and apart from simple remedies I wouldn't recommend anyone to treat herself.'

'I started HRT when I was 51 because I was suffering crippling depression and began to get the most terrible cramp-like back pains. I had to have painkillers and anti-inflammatories, but they didn't touch the pain. It got so bad I was literally crying. The doctor sent me for X-rays and other tests and couldn't find anything. He said it couldn't be the HRT. In the end I was convinced it must be the HRT so I came off it. At that point the back pain disappeared, but the menopausal symptoms returned with a vengeance. I had hot flushes, sweats and vaginal dryness. Then last December I had the most crashing depression. I didn't know what to do, so I returned to the doctor, who

113

suggested I should try a lower dose HRT patch. Within a couple of weeks the back pain came back. The doctor rang the drug company to see if it was a recognized side-effect, and discovered that, though it is rare, they are beginning to see cases. It's muscular cramp. This time I took it into my own hands and came off the HRT.

'The depression came back, so I went to see a homoeopathic practitioner. I told him "I feel so bad I want to pull all my skin off." He prescribed lachesis – which comes from snake venom. For two days I had the most dreadful depression [a common sign that a remedy is working] but since then the depression has vanished and I have been all right, though I still get night sweats. They are a nuisance but I can cope. I still get vaginal dryness, round about the time my period would have been due, but it's not unmanageable.'

JENNIFER, 55

OTHER ALTERNATIVE THERAPIES

Finding the right therapy or therapies to suit you can be a way of caring for yourself – something women often find hard to do. Other therapies worth exploring include massage and aromatherapy – both good for general relaxation and beating stress; acupuncture, which is said to help rebalance the system and improve energy levels; and reflexology. You can find out more about all these therapies in my own book *Alternative Health Care for Women*.

Self-help

BEATING FLUSHES AND SWEATS

HRT is effective at curing flushes and sweats, but there are several things you can do yourself to combat them.

Stay Cool

Getting tense, anxious or embarrassed actually makes flushes worse. They are much less noticeable than you think. When you feel a flush coming on, relax and consciously loosen your shoulders, breathe slowly and as deeply as feels comfortable, and sit still until the flush has passed.

Some women find it helpful to bite the bullet and admit to friends and family that they are suffering hot flushes.

Vitamin E

Some women find vitamin E helpful in combating sweats and flushes. Start with 200 iu a day for a month. If there is no improvement step up the dose to 300 or 400 iu, and if there is still no improvement increase the dose to 500, but don't go over 600 iu a day, except on the advice of a qualified nutritional practitioner. When you have found the lowest level that works stick to it. Do bear in mind that high doses of vitamins act in exactly the same way as drugs (i.e. they have a pharmacological effect), so use them cautiously. If you can afford it it's a good idea to see a qualified nutritional practitioner, who has practice in prescribing food supplements who will be able to tailor the dose to suit you. Vitamin E is not recommended if you suffer diabetes, rheumatic heart disease or high blood-pressure. It's also not known whether it has an effect on the risk of breast cancer.

Ginseng

Ginseng comes from the root of a plant used in traditional medicine as a general stimulant and tonic. It is classed as an 'adaptogen' – that is, a remedy that works by nourishing the body to help cope with stress. As well as hot flushes it is said to be good for loss of sex drive and general debility. However, Kitty Campion in *A Woman's Herbal* warns: 'It should not be given to those . . . suffering from high blood-pressure or nervous tension or anxiety, nor to women with menstrual irregularities. It should never be taken with anything containing caffeine.' For long-term use she suggests a dose of 400–800 mg of the dried root daily. There are several different types of ginseng: Asiatic ginseng (*Panax*), Siberian ginseng (*Eleutherococcus senticosus*) and American ginseng (*Panax quinquefolium*). The Siberian and American varieties are said to be stronger than the Asiatic. Opinions differ as to which is the best quality, and some products include equal parts of the three varieties.

Other herbal remedies for flushes include:

- Taking motherwort and life root, which act on the nervous system (a bit like herbal beta-blockers).
- Cutting down on stimulants: cigarettes, coffee, tea, alcohol, and spicy foods such as curries, as all can trigger flushing.

Naturopath Leon Chaitow suggests the following regime for combating flushes:

- 400 iu vitamin E (with 50 mc of selenium) twice daily
- 1 g vitamin C twice daily
- 1 high-potency vitamin B tablet (containing at least 50 mg of each of the main B vitamins)

INSOMNIA

As we've seen earlier, lack of sleep can be a side-effect of hot flushes. However, once you are awake the troubles of the world can descend upon you, making further sleep impossible. Treatment is two-pronged: first, do what you can to alleviate flushes (see above), secondly pay attention to what experts call sleep hygiene – your bedtime routines, and what you do when you wake in the night.

- Cut out coffee, tea, cigarettes, sugar and alcohol, all of which can interfere with peaceful sleep.
- Make sure you are really tired before you turn in. Get some exercise during the day.
- Wind down slowly at the end of the day. Learn to relax and

practise your relaxation routine in bed. Breathe deeply and slowly, concentrating on the out breath. Tense and relax muscles in turn: arms, neck, shoulders, face, eyes, stomach, back, legs.

- Have a warm milky drink, or an herbal tea such as chamomile before bedtime. Calcium is nature's natural tranquillizer, so making sure you get plenty in your diet will not only benefit your bones but could make for sweeter sleep, too.
- A relaxing massage will help prepare you for sleep.
- If you wake in the night don't try too hard to get back to sleep. Tell yourself 'sleep will come when it is ready' and 'relaxing in bed is almost as good'. If intrusive thoughts threaten to keep you awake, let them go; visualizing a pleasant scene instead, or repeating a word or mantra beneath your breath every few seconds.

DRY VAGINA

There are many alternative methods of alleviating the pain and discomfort of a dry vagina. A diet high in vitamins and minerals (especially the ones mentioned above) is helpful. Plants with an oestrogenic effect (see Herbal Help, page 109) can be used as teas, in salads, or taken as prescribed by a practitioner. Herbal practitioners may also prescribe herbs in gel or douche form. However, although they are less likely to produce the unwelcome side-effects of oestrogen, they are also slower to work.

The authors of the *Encyclopedia of Natural Medicine* recommend:

- B-complex vitamins, 100 mg a day
- Vitamin E, 400 iu a day
- Topical vitamin E cream
- Herbal treatment with phytoestrogenic herbs

Ginseng is used to combat dry vagina in Finland, Russia, China and Japan. However, the authors of *Menopause: A Time for Positive Change* caution: 'It mimics the hormone oestrogen . . . but no one knows if it also mimics the tendency of oestrogen to encourage the growth of cancerous cells or cysts.' They also name swollen and painful breasts and vaginal bleeding as possible side-effects of taking ginseng.

Practise contracting and releasing the muscles of the pelvic floor (the ones you use to control urinating and defecating, and which you can feel contracting when you have an orgasm), as this helps improve circulation to the pelvic region and maintains its elasticity.

Making love and masturbation can also exercise the pelvic floor muscles and improve lubrication – as well as being enjoyable! Make sure you are fully aroused before penetration. *KY* jelly (available from chemists) helps lubrication. Another product, *Replens*, helps rehydrate the tissues of the vagina by causing them to retain natural moisture.

OSTEOPOROSIS

Although osteoporosis is partly a matter of genetic make-up, it's quite clear that it is at least partly a disease of our lifestyle. A diet high in protein and phosphates and low in calcium and other trace minerals, combined with an inactive lifestyle and habits such as smoking and drinking can put you at risk. HRT can help prevent the disease, as we've seen, but there are other things you can do to cut your risk.

A huge debate is going on within the medical profession about the value of calcium and exercise in both the prevention and treatment of osteoporosis. As I explained earlier, there are two parts to the osteoporosis equation: your peak bone mass – the time of your bones' greatest strength and density (around the age of 30 to 35), and the rate at which you lose bone. It used to be thought that exercise was only valuable in strengthening bone during early life. However, more recent studies have shown that exercise can help to build bone – no matter how old you are. Other reliable studies have shown that taking calcium supplements can help, too. However, while these measures may be enough to prevent osteoporosis in those at low risk, women who are already showing signs of the disease need medical treatment.

Once you are over 35 you need about 1 gram of calcium a day, and after the menopause you need 1.5 grams a day. Vitamin D, produced by exposure to the sun and found in foods such as oily fish, eggs, fortified cereals and margarines, is necessary to enable the body to absorb calcium properly. If you do decide to take a supplement, make allowances for the fact that you will be getting some calcium from your diet and go for a supplement with 1 to 1.2 grams of calcium.

The problem is that the absorption and retention of calcium is governed by a complex interplay of hormones. As with all therapies, orthodox or alternative, there are risks as well as benefits. Calcium comes in different forms, and some types have been shown to increase the risk of developing kidney stones. The best type both for absorption and to avoid this problem seems to be calcium citrate. It's best to consult a nutritional therapist so that the dose can be prescribed according to your needs.

A diet of the type outlined above is good – make sure you include plenty of calcium-rich foods. Avoid strict dieting; if you need to lose weight do so gradually and avoid yo-yo dieting, which can also raise blood-pressure and so put you at greater risk of heart disease. Eating more than 15 per cent of your calories as protein promotes calcium loss from the bones, so go easy on the meat. Oily fish, preferably ones with their bones such as sardines and anchovies, is rich in vitamin D and calcium.

Calcium is not the only mineral vital to the building of bone. Recent research has focussed on the role of magnesium. People with osteoporosis have lower magnesium levels than those without the disease. This is thought to be due to the complex interplay of magnesium with the hormones that govern bone growth. A high intake of dairy foods fortified with vitamin D has been found to reduce magnesium absorption.

Vitamin B_6, folic acid and vitamin B_{12} may also help prevent osteoporosis. A shortage of these vitamins results in higher levels

Bone Builders

Foods rich in calcium:
Spinach, kale, watercress, greens, parsley, yoghurt, buttermilk, cheese, sesame seeds, tahini, nuts, canned fish with their bones (such as salmon, sardines and anchovies), corn tortillas, tofu, molasses

Foods rich in magnesium:
Poultry, fish, nuts, milk, honey, green vegetables, wholemeal flour, brown rice, Brewer's yeast

Foods rich in vitamin B_6:
Liver, oily fish, wheatgerm, walnuts, avocados, bananas, cabbage, leafy green vegetables

Foods rich in vitamin B_{12}:
Kidney, liver, eggs, herrings, mackerel, cottage cheese

Foods rich in folic acid:
Leafy green vegetables, bananas, liver, kidney, citrus fruits

Foods rich in vitamin K:
Turnips, greens, broccoli, cabbage, lettuce, liver, green tea, cereals

of an amino acid called homocystein, which is thought to interfere with collagen formation.

Vitamin K, found in green leafy vegetables, has also been suggested as one of the protective factors of a vegetarian diet. This vitamin is needed for the formation of a bone protein called osteocalcin, which helps hold calcium in place within the bone. A shortage of vitamin K could lead to weaker bones due to inadequate osteocalcin levels.

HEART DISEASE
The diet outlined on page 103 has been shown to lower the risk of heart disease – partly due to the high amounts of fruit and

vegetables. Increasing evidence is mounting that the so-called anti-oxidant vitamins – beta carotene (which is converted into vitamin A in the body – vitamin C and vitamin E, all found in fruit and vegetables, help protect against the development of heart disease. They work by 'mopping up' free radicals – the destructive molecules that are released in the body and which can damage the cells. In one study, people with low levels of vitamin E showed a dramatically increased risk of developing angina.

You should also aim to include fish on the menu at least twice a week, which cuts meat consumption and replaces harmful saturated fats with beneficial unsaturated ones. White fish is low in fat and high in vitamins and minerals. Oily fish is especially good because it is rich in a group of polyunsaturates called omega-3 fatty acids, which have been proved to make the blood less sticky and less likely to clot.

Even moderate exercise has been shown to reduce the risk of heart attacks and strokes.

BREAST HEALTH

Because breast cancer is so common following the menopause, whether or not you have taken or are taking HRT it's vital to do everything you can to keep your breasts healthy. Keep an eye on your breasts and note any changes in their shape, position, colour, texture and the appearance of the nipples. Make sure you go for regular breast screening/mammographic checks once you reach 50.

Other factors which have been reported to help keep the breasts healthy include:

● A low-fat diet
   Women in parts of the world where a low-fat diet (of the type described on page 103) is consumed have lower rates of breast cancer, though this has recently been questioned. The reason seems to be that obesity and a high-fat intake affect the way our bodies deal with and store oestrogen.

- Cutting down on coffee, tea, and cola drinks
  These drinks contain chemicals called methylxanthines, which have been linked to higher levels of benign breast disease (lumpy, painful breasts), which in turn have been linked with a greater risk of breast cancer.
- Eating your greens
  Certain vegetables of the cruciferous group – such as turnips, cabbage and cress – have been shown to have a protective effect against breast cancer.
- Stepping up your beta carotene intake
  Beta carotene is found in carrots, red peppers, apricots and other red and yellow fruits (see page 105).
- Cutting down on alcohol (see page 106).
- Taking Evening Primrose Oil
  EPO has been shown in several studies to reduce breast pain and lumpiness. Take three 500-mg capsules twice a day.
- Eating soya beans
  One study showed that women who ate a diet high in soya beans had a lower risk of breast cancer.

As you can see, there are plenty of things you can do to help yourself stay fit and well after the menopause. Looking after yourself can give you a feeling of control over your life – something many women say is lacking after the menopause. Even if you do decide to opt for HRT, the measures outlined in this chapter will enhance your health so that you are in the best possible position to resist any side-effects.

CHAPTER SEVEN

Where Do We Go from Here?

Conventional wisdom has it that the change of life is a period of turmoil: of hot flushes, night sweats, moodiness, misery and waning sexual desire. But conventional wisdom is not always right. In every culture there are stress points, situations that are seen as threatening and which, therefore, predispose us to anxiety and increased sensitivity to physical and mental discomforts. In our society, growing old and the loss of youth threaten us with loss of identity, so it's hardly surprising that the menopause is one such stress point. Much play is made of the awfulness of the menopause, but, as we have seen, while fundamental physical and mental changes do take place, if we understand what is happening and can prepare for it it doesn't always have to be agonizing.

A parallel can be made with the turbulent teens. Psychologists use the term 'puberty' to describe the physical and physiological (internal, hormonal) changes that convert children into reproductive beings, and the term 'adolescence' to describe the emotional and psychological growth that take place.

Perhaps a similar distinction should be made between terms 'the menopause' and 'the change of life'. The menopause comprises a series of physical and physiological changes that convert women from reproductive beings into non-reproductive ones. It is a time when the ovaries stop releasing eggs, when oestrogen levels fall, when the vagina becomes dryer. Secondary sexual characteristics are also affected (the breasts may become smaller and more flaccid, pubic hair becomes more scanty). HRT can help with some of the troublesome physical symptoms these changes bring about and may help with some of the mental ones.

The change of life, on the other hand, refers to the much more hazy process of growing older, both physically and psychologically, and – given the symbolic significance we attach to the ability to reproduce as women, and the many life changes that may also be taking place at this time – it can take much longer than the menopause itself. What HRT cannot do is prevent us from growing older. The change can involve a sense of loss, but if we allow ourselves to experience that loss it can also be a time of positive growth, when we can move on to a new future free of the shackles of biology. Germaine Greer's book, *The Change: Women, Ageing and the Menopause* addresses these points. Ms Greer is violently against HRT and the book doesn't make comfortable reading. It does highlight, however, some of the issues that make the menopause such a difficult transition – and for that reason it makes valuable reading for anyone entering or going through the change.

All cultures have methods of relieving the distress of the various life transitions. In our technological society, we tend to put our faith in pharmacological relief, in much the same way as we turn to drugs to relieve the pain of labour. Other types of help tend to be dismissed as unproven, or ignored altogether. Yet sharing the experience with others, or trying herbal and homoeopathic remedies, are ways of easing the pain of the menopause that can help women to feel active participants in the process of menopause rather than putting them in the passive role of patients.

At the time of writing, the jury is still out on HRT. On one side are the doctors – and, it has to be said, the millions of women who feel they have benefited from the treatment. They admit that yes, there are still some question marks over the risks of breast cancer and uterine bleeding – but we still don't know precisely what these are; and yes, HRT does have some side-effects – but these can usually be sorted out when treatment is tailored to the individual. These people believe that, on balance, the benefits outweigh the risks. On the other side are the disaffected, who feel HRT hasn't helped them, those who say that the social and emotional aspects of the menopause have been medicalized, and other voices of dissent, who say that we still don't know enough about the drug to prescribe it on a wide scale.

If you think HRT might be for you, you should – as I have emphasized again and again – choose it with a full knowledge of the pros and cons. You must recognize that it's not a panacea for all the stresses and challenges that face women as they negotiate the mid-life transition. The benefits of HRT are undeniable, but, as we have seen, the risks are as yet neither clearly nor totally defined, and are unlikely to be for some time.

Research into HRT is continuing. Within the next few years, hopefully, we will have more answers to some of the questions raised about the treatment. In the meantime, scientists are working on several promising new developments. These include:

- New types of progestogens with fewer side-effects than those used at present.
- New combinations of oestrogen and progestogen which avoid the nuisance of withdrawal bleeds.
- A nasal spray containing the hormone calcitonin which can stop bone loss and increase bone mass.
- New forms of nonhormonal vaginal lubricants.
- New methods of delivering progestogen such as a vaginal ring or IUD that can be left in place long term.

On the alternative front, as natural therapies are beginning to be taken more seriously the opportunities for exploring different avenues of treatment are increasing, too. Many doctors are becoming more knowledgeable about alternative and comp-lementary therapies, and some are even offering treatment as part of their medical practice.

One thing is certain: the controversy surrounding HRT is unlikely to go away. In the meantime it is vital to keep up to date with the latest reports on HRT.

Unfortunately this is far from easy. All too many doctors fall into one of two camps: the unreservedly enthusiastic, who believe all women should have their wombs whipped out after they have finished childbearing and go on HRT, and the cautious or uninterested, who refuse to recognize the potential advantages of treatment on the grounds that these advantages are unproven.

The press, as I mentioned in the Introduction, is only likely to concern itself with the most lurid headlines. If you read about HRT in a popular newspaper, try to find the source and check it out to make sure you have the facts behind the headlines.

If you are not happy with your doctor, ask for a second opinion – or even change doctors. You can also make the menopause clinic work for you. It's no good complaining that such clinics are HRT production lines if you don't make it clear that you want alternatives. If you don't want a prescription for HRT, say so. You can use the facilities such as bone scanning, nutritional counselling and advice without necessarily accepting a prescription for a drug that you don't feel happy with. The best menopause clinics work holistically, they look at you in the context of your entire lifestyle and circumstances and attempt to help you decide what is right for you.

In the last resort it comes down to deciding what is an acceptable level of risk for you. As one woman said:

'I had such a bad menopause that my life was hell.
Then I took HRT and after about three days the
difference was dramatic, I felt normal again. Why
should I go back to hell once I've found a way out?'

That said, HRT isn't right for everybody. Like childbirth, the menopause can be a powerful symbol of lack of control: all of a sudden your body is behaving in an untoward and unpredictable way. For some women taking HRT can be a means to wrench back that control.

For others the opposite is the case: taking HRT means putting themselves under medical control. For such women self-help and alternative therapies may be a more potent way of taking charge of their lives.

> 'As soon as I started taking the homoeopathic remedy I got my brain back. I decided to give up my job. For a while I had wanted to get out; when I got my brain back I fathomed what I wanted to do. I couldn't stand the thought of doing what I was doing until I was 60. Now I am enjoying life again. Homoeopathy put me back in charge.'
>
> RUTH, 45

The choice is yours.

Further Reading

The Change: Women, Ageing and the Menopause, Germaine Greer, (Hamish Hamilton, 1991).

HRT: Your Questions Answered, Malcolm Whitehead and Val Godfree, (Churchill Livingstone, 1992).
(Although aimed at doctors and basically pro-HRT, this book contains much useful information on the various studies done.)

Menopause: A Time for Positive Change, Judi Fairlie, Jayne Nelson and Ruth Popplestone (Javelin, 1988).

Your Menopause: Prepare Now for a Positive Future, Myra Hunter (Pandora, 1990).

Useful Addresses

UK

Amarant Trust
Grant House
56–60 St John Street
London EC1M 4DT
Tel. 071–490 1644
Produce an information pack (£5 and s.a.e. at time of writing).
The Trust also has a list of menopause clinics.

National Osteoporosis Society
PO Box 10
Radstock
Bath BA3 3YP
Tel. 0761 432472

Can send you a list of hospitals with bone scanners in your area
as well as other information (please send s.a.e. and a second-
class stamp).

Women's Health Concern
17 Earl's Terrace
London W8
Tel. 071–602 6669

Women's Health and Reproductive Rights Information Centre (WHRRIC)
52 Featherstone Street
London EC1Y 8RT
Tel. 071–251 6580

Produce leaflets on the menopause, hysterectomy and HRT. Send s.a.e. for full list of leaflets and prices. Also offers information on a range of women's health topics, and can give you contact numbers for local women's groups.

ALTERNATIVE THERAPIES

All Hallows Natural Health Centre
Tel. 071–283 8908

British Homoeopathic Association
27a Devonshire Street
London W1

The Hale Clinic
7 Park Crescent
London W1N 3HE
Tel. 071–637 3377/071–631 0156

Institute for Complementary Medicine
PO Box 194
London SE16 1QZ
Tel. 071–237 5165

National Institute of Medical Herbalists
9 Palace Gate
Exeter
EX1 1JA
Tel. 0392 426022

Society of Homoeopaths
2 Artizan Road
Northampton NN1 4HU
Tel. 0604 21400

Women's Natural Health Centre
1 Hillside
Highgate Road
London NW5
Tel. 071–482 3293

MENOPAUSE CLINICS
(addresses correct at time of writing)

This is just a selection. For local information contact your GP, local hospital gynaecology department, Well Woman or Family Planning clinic. Alternatively, write or phone The Amarant Trust or WHRRIC.

NHS Services
NHS menopause clinics usually require a letter from your doctor.

ENGLAND

Birmingham and Midland Hospital for Women
Showall Green Lane
Sparkhill
Birmingham
Tel. 021–772 1101

Good Hope Hospital
Rectory Road
Sutton Coldfield
West Midlands
Tel. 021–378 2211

Annie Wood Resource Centre
129 Alma Way
Lozells
Birmingham
Tel. 021–554 7137

Family Planning Clinic
Morley Street
Brighton
Tel. 0273 696011

Family Planning Clinic
Countess of Chester Hospital
Liverpool Road
Chester
Tel. 0244 365000

Well Woman Centre
Eleanor Street
Grimsby
Tel. 0472 354113
(Counselling and advice only)

Princess Royal Hospital
Salthouse Road
Hull
Tel. 0482 701151

Menopause Clinic
The Women's Hospital
Catharine Street
Liverpool L8 7NJ
Tel. 051–709 1000

Bloomsbury Menopause Clinic
Elizabeth Garret Anderson Hospital for Women
144 Euston Road
London NW1
Tel. 071–387 2501

Department of Medicine
Newcastle General Hospital
Westgate Road
Newcastle upon Tyne NE4 6BE
Tel. 091–273 8811

NORTHERN IRELAND

Belfast Maternity Hospital
Grosvenor Road
Belfast BT12 6BA
Tel. 0232 240503

SCOTLAND

Ward 42/43
Aberdeen Royal Infirmary
Foresterhill
Aberdeen
Tel. 0224 681818, ext. 53470

Bone Metabolism Unit
Western Infirmary
Glasgow G11 6NT
Tel. 041–339 8822

Stobhill Hospital
Balornock Road
Glasgow
Tel. 041–558 0111

WALES

Gynaecology Department
Singleton Hospital
Sketty
Swansea SA2 8QA
Tel. 0792 205666

Private Clinics

ENGLAND

The Amarant Centre
South Cheshire Private Hospital
Leighton
Crewe CW1 4QP
Tel. 0270 500411

The Amarant Centre
Churchill Clinic
80 Lambeth Road
London SE1 7PW
Tel. 071–401 3855

BUPA Hospital Portsmouth
Bartons Road
Havant
Hants PO9 5NP
Tel. 0705 454511

REPUBLIC OF IRELAND

Dr Mary Short
59 Synge Street
Dublin 8
Tel. 780712

USA

Women's Health Advisory Service
PO Box 31000
Phoenix
AZ 85046

The American Foundation of Traditional Chinese Medicine
1280 Columbus Avenue
Suite 302
San Francisco, CA 94133
Tel: (415) 776 0502

Center for Medical Consumers
237 Thompson Street
New York, NY 10012
Tel: (212) 674 7105

Santa Cruz Women's Health Center
250 Locust Street
Santa Cruz, CA 95060
Tel: (408) 427 3500

Vitamin Suppliers:

Natren Ltd.
12142 Huston Street
North Hollywood
CA 91607

Australia

Women's Health Advisory Service
PO Box 1096
Bankstown 2200

Women's Health Care Association
92 Thomas Street
West Perth
WA 6005

Australian Natural Therapists' Association
PO Box 522
Sutherland
New South Wales 2232
Tel: (02) 521 2063

Healthsharing Women
318 Little Bourke Street
Melbourne
Victoria 3000
Tel: (03) 663 4457

Women's Health Information Resource Collective
653 Nicholson Street
Carlton North
Victoria 3054
Tel: (03) 387 8702

Women's Health Information Centre
Royal Women's Hospital
132 Grattan Street
Carlton
Victoria 3053
Tel: (03) 344 2007/2199

Index

NATURAL HORMONE HEALTH
Drug-free ways to balance your life

ARABELLA MELVILLE

Hormones can play havoc with your life, whatever your age. Indeed, fluctuating and imbalanced hormones can be the cause of such disruptions to your life as premenstrual syndrome, hot flushes, mood swings, period pain, cravings, osteoporosis and weight problems.

Hormone treatment of various sorts is growing, but there *are* alternatives to drugs and surgical intervention.

Arabella Melville, a pharmacologist and health writer, examines all these options from a holistic standpoint, explaining how a diet incorporating the right minerals, vitamins and fats, together with sensible exercise, relaxation and other natural therapies can free you completely from all hormone-related problems.

NATURAL HORMONE HEALTH	0 7225 2815 9	£4.99	☐
BREAST AWARENESS	0 7225 2789 6	£4.99	☐
CYSTITIS	0 7225 2693 8	£3.99	☐
FIBROIDS	0 7225 2801 9	£4.99	☐
PELVIC INFLAMMATORY DISEASE & CHLAMYDIA	0 7225 2608 3	£3.99	☐
OSTEOPOROSIS	0 7225 2509 5	£3.99	☐
SMEAR TESTS	0 7225 2500 1	£3.99	☐
BLADDER PROBLEMS	0 7225 2508 7	£3.99	☐
THRUSH	0 7225 2503 6	£3.99	☐

All these books are available from your local bookseller or can be ordered direct from the publishers.

To order direct just tick the titles you want and fill in the form below:

NAME: _____

ADDRESS: _____

_____

_____ POSTCODE: _____

Send to: Thorsons Mail Order, Dept 3, HarperCollins*Publishers*, Westerhill Road, Bishopbriggs, Glasgow G64 2QT.
Please enclose a cheque or postal order or your authority to debit your Visa/Access account —

CREDIT CARD NO: _____

EXPIRY DATE: _____

SIGNATURE: _____

— up to the value of the cover price plus:
UK & BFPO: Add £1.00 for the first book and 25p for each additional book ordered.

Overseas orders including Eire: Please add £2.95 service charge. Books will be sent by surface mail but quotes for airmail despatches will be given on request.

24 HOUR TELEPHONE ORDERING SERVICE FOR ACCESS/VISA CARDHOLDERS — TEL: **041 772 2281.**